Crossing Out The Emperor

Michael Black

chipmunkapublishing
the mental health publisher

All rights reserved, no part of this publication may be reproduced by any means, electronic, mechanical photocopying, documentary, film or in any other format without prior written permission of the publisher.

>Published by
>Chipmunkapublishing
>PO Box 6872
>Brentwood
>Essex CM13 1ZT
>United Kingdom

http://www.chipmunkapublishing.com

Copyright © Michael Black 2011

ISBN   978-1-84991-671-4

Chipmunkapublishing gratefully acknowledge the support of Arts Council England.

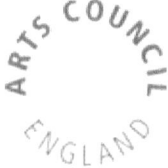

Author Biography

Michael Black was born in England in 1962. He studied literature and history at York University before completing a doctorate at Cambridge University in South African studies, and has spent his adult life fascinated with exploring the territory at which history ends and literature begins (or vice-versa). His stage plays (www.mwblack.co.uk), performed in Edinburgh, York, Cardiff, Manchester and London as well as in Eastern Europe, frequently give witness to this, as does *Crossing Out The Emperor*, his first novel. Of this he is convinced; the real territory of creation is myth.

Crossing Out The Emperor

Foreword

This novel has nothing to do with mental health, but everything to do with proving my sanity. My intention in publication is to prove I can write outside the subject of mental health, and yet at the same time I suppose to implicitly argue that there is no subject that is not *within* the field of mental health. Why so? Because this novel represents, apart from my stage plays, what I was writing during the years I was living the experiences of *Angels, Cleopatra And Psychosis* and *Leonardo, Romancia And Ra*, but stands quite apart from them.

Within this novel there is no mention or discussion of psychiatry at all, but at the same time, a great deal of this novel was written whilst I was in and out of psychiatric wards 1994-2001. Its completion represents my determination to escape the psychiatric system for good and all.

But what is psychiatry? *Psychiatry is extremity*. And this is a novel of extremity, the extremity of Beethoven's "fiery, active temperament" in love and Napoleon at his military nadir of 1812. And I think it can be argued that all forms of personal extremity are forms of madness. Or rather, *the mind in extremity occupies a world of madness*, that is to say, of experience unreachable to most other, so-called *sane* people.

Sane people are *boring*, and the great or remarkable are never classifiable as one or the other.

Napoleon on his retreat from Russia in the chapter *Incognito* is quite clearly mad in the sense of being deluded, and his vast schemes to be the Emperor of Europe are in fact typical of what a psychiatrist today would refer to as the *grandiose thinking* of a manic depressive. Further, Josephine speaks of the "unspoken malady that [still] consumes him." Is that malady physical or mental?

And Kay Redfield Jamison in *Touched With Fire* quotes psychiatric evidence that Beethoven's famed eccentricity at least bordered, if did not cross, the line of the psychotic, although personally I can find no evidence of this in his music. Quite the contrary, but then I've only ever met one psychiatrist with any musical interests! *But what is hypomania and what is joy?* In the discussion of the *Ode to Joy* in the chapter *Heiligenstadt*, I hope you will remember that question.

A female pianist friend of mine, obsessed, as I am, by Beethoven's 32 piano sonatas, read the manuscript of this novel and quite blatantly asked me if I "knew the spirit of Ludwig [van Beethoven.]" So I said "yes, I do." She said "so do I, but I thought it only happened to musicians" (I am not one.) The following conversation between us was private...

Or rather almost. Because of course Ludwig was there. I completed this novel in 2001, but during the eight years of writing *Crossing Out The Emperor*, I came to know his spirit very well, he just lived in my kitchen and was available to be talked to at any time I liked. He slept on the floor, got in the way, and hummed to himself incessantly. Hence my inside line on the Beethoven subject to some extent, whatever the research I also did, which was very necessary (Beethoven, when asked the details of his life and compositions, 200 years after his death, had forgotten a great deal himself!).

So this is a book that bears testimony to the existence of spirits just as much as my two former books for Chipmunka, and in that sense, naturally finishes a trilogy. What a roller coaster spirit ride I've had! I've met Michelangelo, Leonardo da Vinci, Queen Cleopatra, Romancia, Delacroix, Géricault, the Sun God Ra, and a few more I didn't like I'd rather not name. But Ludwig was the one who could calm me, the one who knew me best when all is said and done... Perhaps Ludwig is the one I love the most...

As will be discovered upon the reading, I wrote this novel to reclaim Beethoven's love life for him, and, in the composition, quickly discovered it required framing by contemporary events. And the big contemporary event of Beethoven's life was Napoleon.

So I quickly realised I was writing a historical novel, and went back to the founder of the *genre*, Sir Walter Scott, for inspiration. Naturally ambitious, my self-appointed aim was to "re-invent the historical novel" by combining the scholarship I learnt doing my doctorate with history and romance. I don't know if I've succeeded, but guess what? Sir Walter Scott's spirit turned up as well, and, since I'd never written a novel before, proved invaluable in his help and inspiration along the way. So much so, he directed me to his essentially un-read *Life Of Napoleon* (1827), from which short parts of the chapter *Incognito* are essentially lifted.

Scott's influence on me was almost as calming as that of the Beethoven I came to know so well, although more cerebral. So he too must be added to the number of spirits I have met. Psychiatrically of course, I then made a rod for my own back by one day mentioning to my psychiatrist at the time (their numbers have changed like those in a lottery) that I was "having dream sex with the ancient queen Cleopatra by night and talking to Sir Walter Scott by day" only to find, very frighteningly, that I was then urgently considered as a candidate for long term locked up care! But that is not the point. The point is that psychiatrists don't like people who hear voices, and I think voices are spirits who the hearers haven't identified yet (and perhaps never will.) And there are of course evil spirits as well as good spirits, as *Angels, Cleopatra And Psychosis* clearly documents.

But as I said, this is not a book about psychiatry. It is however a book, since I have admitted to spirit interventions, that was written in moods psychiatrists would document as psychotic. In other words, as ever, psychiatrists get it wrong. *There are more things in heaven and earth,* Dr. Kraepelin [the definer of schizophrenia], *than are dreamt of in your philosophy…*

I could go on with this spirit story of mine. Because of course, setting out as I did to reclaim Ludwig's love life, it proved no surprise when some of his lovers mentioned in the novel then turned up too. So suddenly my house was full of girls! Great fun! But I'm not going to say which ones before you've read the novel, because it would ruin the story…

One last thing. Concerning the female pianist friend of mine, she once visited Beethoven's grave in Vienna, and found a ring on the grave with the initials "AB" marked upon it. But that will make more sense to you when you've read the whole book…

Michael Black

For my Family

I am above all a just man, *Napoleon, 1804*

Never again will a story be told as if it is the only one, *John Berger*

It's all moonshine next to the education of the heart, *Sir Walter Scott*

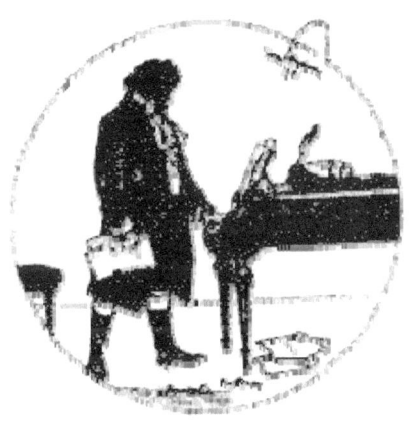

Malheuresement les génies médiocres sont condamnés à imiter les défauts des grands maîtres sans en apprécier les beautés: de là le mal que Michel-Ange fait à la peinture, Shakespeare à l'art dramatique et que Beethoven fait nos jours à la musique.

Unfortunately, mediocre talents are condemned to imitate the faults of the great masters without achieving their virtues: hence the harm Michelangelo does to painting, Shakespeare to drama, and nowadays Beethoven to music.

(From Beethoven's Notebooks, 1816, source unknown)

For my Family

I am above all a just man, *Napoleon, 1804*

Never again will a story be told as if it is the only one, *John Berger*

It's all moonshine next to the education of the heart, *Sir Walter Scott*

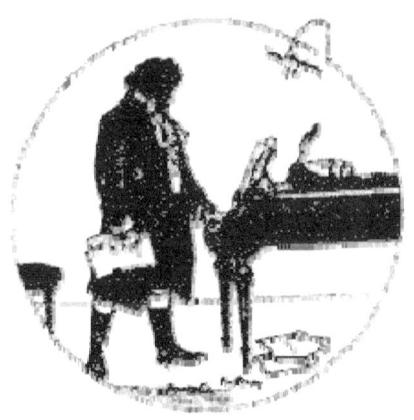

Malheuresement les génies médiocres sont condamnés à imiter les défauts des grands maîtres sans en apprécier les beautés: de là le mal que Michel-Ange fait à la peinture, Shakespeare à l'art dramatique et que Beethoven fait nos jours à la musique.

Unfortunately, mediocre talents are condemned to imitate the faults of the great masters without achieving their virtues: hence the harm Michelangelo does to painting, Shakespeare to drama, and nowadays Beethoven to music.

(From Beethoven's Notebooks, 1816, source unknown)

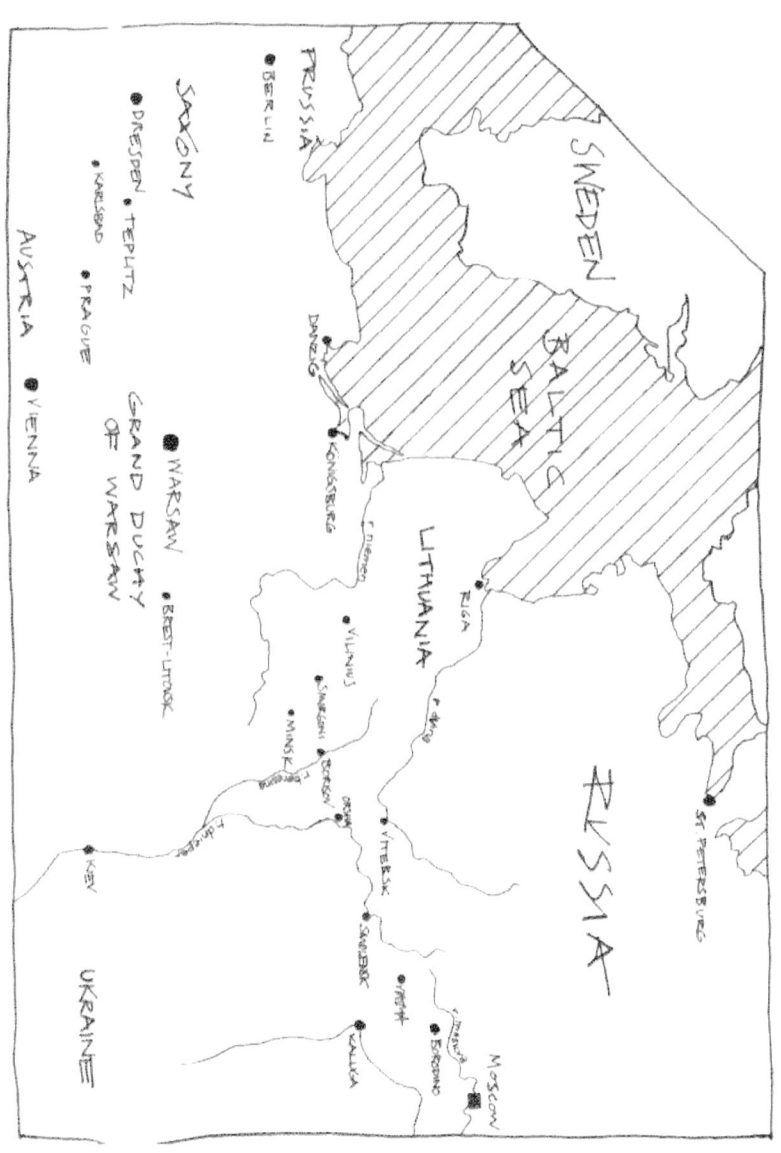

Crossing Out The Emperor

Michael Black

A WOMAN SCORNED

Humiliation! Standing in the throne room whilst the Emperor read out his reasoning for the divorce. And most of the bitching dog kennel of his family were at his side, in full silk and robes, their stone faces concealing their delight that the struggle of thirteen years was ending with the triumph of their will over my own. How often silk socks conceal eczema! There stood Louis the mad King of Holland, Caroline the Queen of Naples, Jérôme the King of Westphalia, and Pauline the pretty but dim-witted Princess Borghese, together through the second born of their number the most crowned family in Europe. Madame Mère, the prize bitch that bred them stayed away, but I knew she'd be smiling in secret even as my marriage vanished before me. Coward, coward, coward! I could have scratched out her eyes and swallowed them whole, no matter the consequences.

The Emperor coughed. Though dressed as ever in his beloved dark green uniform of a colonel in the Chasseurs, he looked short and squat. But then he was never impressive deprived of his General's hat. Wiping the sweat from his palms, he concluded by stating his only motive was the good of the state, and then handed me my own statement of agreement. He had written it himself. "With the permission of my august and dear husband, I declare that having no further hope of children who would satisfy the needs of his policy and the interest of France, I am pleased to offer him the greatest proof of attachment and devotion that could be given..."

I was pleased to offer no such thing, but what choice did I have? *Bon-a-parte est Bon-à-rien!* Understand this. The Council of State, each and every one of them appointed by the Emperor himself, found reason to cast doubt over the civil contract of marriage.

The wording was said to be suspect, and with great convenience, no one could find the wooden-legged Monsieur Lecombe who had conducted the ceremony. Such legal invention hardly surprised me, but the ease with which Cardinal Fesch did away with the religious marriage took my breath away. I'd always known the civil ceremony was insufficient for my purpose. That is why, armed with the Pope's insistence, I had contrived the religious marriage prior to the Coronation. Afterwards, I pursued the Cardinal for two whole days before he surrendered to me the certificate of legality. I had clutched it to my bosom knowing full well the security it bestowed; only to find it bestowed nothing! The Cardinal, though he had conducted the ceremony in person, now saw fit to argue it null and void for want of a parish priest. Cambacérès, a most treacherous lawyer, found no evidence that the Emperor had ever granted his consent (to his own wedding!) The gutless Berthier and Talleyrand, so consummate a Foreign Minister he could lie fluently in five languages, suddenly found they had no recollection of having ever been present. Aspersions were cast that I must have forged their signatures of witness, and there was no higher authority than the Cardinal to whom I could resort with my honest grievances. No doubt anticipating his own actions, my newly freed husband had recently confiscated all the Italian Vatican lands and held the Pope prisoner at Savona. *Bon-a-parte est Bon-à-rien!*

So ended the marriage of Josephine to Napoleon on the 16th of December 1809. I had screamed and cried and fainted my protests to no avail save to gain the opinion of crooked doctors that I was over-wrought and unbalanced, accusations that circulate to this day. *What of them?* A forty-six year old obstacle to diplomacy, my life was stripped bare, consoled by nothing save the Elysée for life, the estate of Malmaison in full ownership and three million francs a year. I was not, Cardinal Fesch assured me, even a divorcée, since I had in fact never been married at all but had lived a decade and more in concubinage. A whore for thirteen years! Well, what of it? Enough had whispered it, let those who must spit it spit it publicly at last. I'll be damned if I mourn a reputation amidst this Empire of liars and cheats.

Oh, I'll want for nothing, I grant you that. Napoleon is never mean. His is a kind of absent-minded cruelty born of self-obsession. And, ever an adornment and never alone mighty, neither am I truly fallen. Besides, not even a corrupt Cardinal can steal away empty rhetoric, and so I retain my title. As I sit in these gardens of Malmaison I am still the Empress Josephine. An Empress mark! Whether as wife or concubine, spinster or *une femme libre*, it is a giddy height of fame for Marie-Josèphe-Rose de Tascher de la Pagerie, the sugar planter's daughter from indolent Martinique, a bird of the islands, ambitious for nothing except an ample sufficiency of leisure and gossip. For twenty-five years the maelstrom has picked me up and turned me in its urgent motion. I have survived near shipwrecks; I have cheated the guillotine, thwarted the plots of assassins and lived a life of love and war in full measure. Passion has been constant in its rage around me, and I, of a calmer ilk, have found my life dictated by it daily. Always, always Napoleon! These gardens of Malmaison I planted myself, but the cedar I sit beneath is his. He brought it from Marengo to be planted in celebration of his great victory, and in time it will grow to dominate all. On Martinique my mother called me Yeyette. When I first came to France I signed myself Marie-Rose. It was Napoleon who decided upon Josephine, and as Josephine I now know myself and shall always be known. But now, since the maelstrom has set me down for good and all, I'll speak for myself as well as any, and I'll spare no reputations.

What makes the desires and ambitions of men so puerile? What makes them so vainglorious and deceitful? Oh, I ask no pity and I know I'll receive none. There's many a wronged woman more wronged than me and with less compensation to boot. But marry Napoleon Bonaparte and you find out soon enough. There's nothing more to men than the impregnation of women, and until a man succeeds in that he succeeds in nothing. What haste! No sooner had Napoleon cast me aside, than Talleyrand had a list prepared of seventeen eligible young women, each from a royal house and all with good pedigrees, swelling breasts and child-bearing hips. Such unfulfilled obsession! Oh, I suffer from none myself. Before I met Napoleon I bore two children by marriage to one Alexander, an idling swine and the first of many to christen me whorish. Alexander believed that I had shown favour to most of the French garrison of Martinique and a good many negroes besides (why else would I have bought some their freedom?) Allegations so beyond all reason that even the crusty judges of Châtelet, hardly strangers to whoring themselves, saw fit to grant me a petition of slander. No matter. But consider the facts! Before turning eighteen, I had already provided Alexander with the son Napoleon has abandoned me for not presenting to him! No thanks from Napoleon for incapacities I believe to be his own, and no love or comfort from Alexander before him. How easy men find it to call a woman a whore and how difficult for a woman to seem virtuous. Alexander was no sooner disgracing my name than he was parading his own concubine, that slut Madame de Longpré, in front of my very mother. I was the whore, but Alexander's of course was a grand passion. I've heard de Longpré could milk men dry with silk gloves on, and I'll not contradict a rumour for want of witness. Consumed by weakness, Alexander invested me with all of his own. No more or no less, a mere copulating infant.

Oh, let it be loudly said, I've had affairs myself. But these are only the stuff of loneliness and pleasure, and most, though I'll not say all, I'd have happily exchanged for a husband who'd spend three parts of a year with his wife in preference to his never-ending campaigns and conquests. No sooner had Napoleon married me he vanished to Italy for ten months, no sooner did he return he vanished again to Egypt for a whole two years! And his only motive for return that I could see was the coup d'état. Campaigns and battles were the rulers of our marriage, and his successes only made such circumstances worse. He took to travelling forever across his dominions in Italy and Germany and Holland, planting his scheming relatives on thrones far and wide. And then, never trusting them to rule, he took to overseeing the entire duties of each and every one of them! Once, when briefly he was in residence with me at Malmaison, so used was he to sleeping beneath the stars that he abandoned our bed for a tent pitched in the gardens! Though he requested it, I did not join him.

And so in truth, though a few brave men have whispered against it, it comes as no surprise to me that he now seeks the conquest of Russia. Where else is there left for him? He'll not settle for some squabble with the British in Spain. It has insufficient scale. One man astride the continent is what he seeks, and so his new Empress in the Tuileries will sit for months and quite possibly years awaiting his return. The sweet and lonely innocent Austrian seventeen-year-old he has taken for his bride will want for nothing save the presence of her spouse. But then perhaps this Marie-Louise, with too ample an arse to be truly elegant (though I say it myself), is much taken with her aggrandisement, and Napoleon is said to be delirious. Happily presented with the son of his desires at last, one Napoleon-Francis, already the King of Rome! Bah! I'll believe none of it. That child is an impostor, the produce of some street girl planted in a royal cradle through dire necessity. Or else the child is from some illicit union Marie-Louise has sown and reaped at the court. I favour the first. A street girls unwanted carry less danger than the illegitimate offspring of a count or duke, or even, Heaven forbid, of one of Napoleon's own marshals! Consider it all! He can disguise to himself his impotence with a forty six year old Empress, but how can the delusion continue when he takes a seventeen year old to his bed? Oh, and I know better than any the duplicity which surrounds him. There are none more desperate for a son than the Emperor. This new marriage (what legality this!) was conducted by proxy, the Emperor in Paris, the bride in Vienna, with her father, the Austrian Emperor himself, leaving her no choice in the matter for fear of French invasion. The pretty union thus completed, I've heard that when Marie-Louise first met her new master, Napoleon immediately took with her to the boudoir where the couple remained a full seven hours. He's a slave to paternity! And Marie-Louise, well! What shock must have confronted her. If stories of her virginity be true, Napoleon is a strange introduction. I'll not believe he abandoned our bed only for want of passion. I could see the changes for myself. There are strange transformations beneath his uniform of that I'm sure.

The greater details escape me, so total became his guarding of his body from my sight. But I lived within the grip of contradiction nonetheless. I refused all doctoring (there is nothing wrong with me!), but still he sent me to take the waters at Aix-les-Bains and Aix-la-Chappelle. When once I humoured his strategic frustrations by suggesting he sought conquest of England only for me to bathe in Bath, he could not even smile! He even insisted I visit the sulphurous springs at

Plombières! In the name of Heaven, sulphur! The very imbibing would have killed any child within me, but I went all the same, for it kept up the pretence that the obstacle to offspring was me, and it follows on, that such a matter was subject to cure. And all the while I witnessed his own withering and pretended, in part for love, that I saw nothing.

Be sure of my witness, for there's more than me privy to the secret. The rumours abound, so multiple did his inconstancy become. Oh, there was no concealment. Napoleon would often brag of his conquests, and of his performance with them (to only the latter was I sceptical.) Though he'll never know it, at times it has even been me who has paid his companions of lust to whisper nothing of what they had seen. How ironic the love of a woman for a man! How little a virtuous woman is ever thanked! For I heard at once the scamperings of singers and actresses around the Tuileries at night, and did at once what I saw fit. I have silenced Madame Grassini of the opera and even comforted Mademoiselle George, who woke me with her running and screaming from what she had seen. I even paid for her reinstatement at the Comedie Francaise, for less than satisfied by her visit; Napoleon had insisted she be sacked.

There's a silent conspiracy of women across Europe, I can venture no other explanation. Each and every one of us who have occupied the Emperor's bed must surely know the truth. We are not blind! But as so often, we pretend to be. And it's not the Mademoiselle Georges' I speak of here. There's no blindness there, only an agreement to stay silent for profit. But even now, I still find myself somehow pretending I do not know, and pretending that others who most certainly do know have no knowledge either. Never forget, at the Coronation, Napoleon saw fit to crown himself, in a single stroke rendering the Pope redundant long before he held him literal prisoner. What a perfect act of self-advancement, and how the self-advancers have come to swarm around him! It is the duplicity of other women that brought me down, women who have found pensions and many other gifts in presenting Napoleon with the male issue of affairs apparently his.

What connivance! I am well aware Napoleon confided his frustrated desire for offspring with his sister Caroline (she mocked great concern as she delighted in telling me). And Caroline, herself concerned at her husband General Murat's barrack liaisons, thus removed the object of his affections, one Eléanore de la Plaigne, by informing this unsurprisingly malleable *femme de boudoir* that she would find more profit with Napoleon himself. The result? Within the year Eléanore was parading the child Léon for all to see, whispering in mock secrecy it was the child of the Emperor whilst a whole idle barracks of officers were eager no doubt to serve her! From this point on, my cards were marked. The next ambitious schemer was Maria Walewska, whose charms were so great Napoleon made no effort of return to see me, nor none to have me visit him for a full year! The wilful Maria had him clutched in Poland. I was powerless and he smitten.

The episode with Eléanore and the offspring Léon had not over concerned me. Though Napoleon sought to keep the matter from me, he made no show of affection for the child, seeming both unconcerned and unconvinced that the boy Léon might be his. But Maria was altogether different. In possession of attractions to make any wife wary, she was also desirous of good service. Locked at eighteen into marriage with a seventy year old count, she was heady with the aphrodisiacs of position Napoleon presented. And I would wager, even a man of Napoleon's decaying condition must seem virile against a septuagenarian. To make matters worse, it was at this time that Napoleon-Charles, the five year old son of my daughter Hortense and Napoleon's brother Louis, was taken from us. My own attempts to prise the Emperor from Maria were thus relegated as I sought to comfort my daughter in Holland. And all plans I had fostered that the Emperor, who had always looked fondly on Napoleon-Charles, would one day consider him as heir were dashed forever. What fecund Jezebels women can be! Maria took her chance, and amidst this background of death and grief duly presented Napoleon with a male off-spring she swore to be his, one Alexandre-Florian.

This time, Napoleon proudly paraded the child as his own, and upon returning to Paris, had Maria entertained in rooms at the Elysée. I date my own decline to be irreversible from this event. Be it true or no, now Napoleon was convinced of his own true manhood, and thus certain the former obstacle had been myself. What grand self-delusion! This child of a curious eighteen year old Countess could have been anyone's! Why so late in this history of illicit fornication had women suddenly come to bear Napoleon children? Why no children by his earlier dalliances with Désirée Clary or Madame Pernon (and doubtless many more besides!) both being women about whom to this day he considers me ignorant?

I eke out my days of loneliness and betrayal, but I wish only for the good of France! Many is the time the truth has been dismissed for being the work of the bitter or the half-deranged, but I am neither, being only saddened and weary at the practice of delusion and falsehood. Throughout I have held my pride, though icily. Being never of great subtlety, Napoleon to this very house has sent both Marie-Louise with her screaming King of Rome, and Maria Walewska with the brat

Alexandre-Florian. He was, he wrote, certain of the pleasure these visits would bestow on me! And so I remarked to both these mothers of less than half my years how sweetly their infants played, and (how could I not say it?) what great resemblance to the Emperor they both bore. Together we took our *déjeuner* and walked the grounds, never speaking of what we all must know, but smiling sweetly with the teeth of sharks. Seldom can the entertainer of a *crèche* have felt such hatred to its young mothers.

To what standards have both men and women sunk! And crowning it all, at this very time Napoleon's greatest romance, the Grande Armée, is assembling at rendezvous' all over the Continent. The greatest military force in history has commenced its march on Russia. It is said 600,000 men are regimented. 200,000 horses and more are commandeered; cattle too for sustenance, the making of two million pairs of boots have occupied every cobbler in France and many beyond (with what mercantile irony the shoemakers of England have supplied their enemy!) Along with the prostitutes and the cooks, the nurses and engineers and cranking artillery, whole chests of forged Russian currency are to be transported. The harlequinade assembles! Once again, the reluctant conscripts, the heroic Imperial Guard, the idealistic and the naive, the ambitious and the venal, the marshals of many battles and the eager officers in search of loot, promotion and glory all seek to expand the Empire of France. The allies of this vast movement this very week entertain the Emperor's entourage at Dresden, in a display of affection so grandiose as to deceive only one so sick as Napoleon himself. To Dresden have come the well-born, the wit and the beauty of Europe. The Kings and Queens of Wurtemberg and Saxony, the Emperor and Empress of Austria, the King of Bavaria with his many duchesses. The Emperor will enter this self-serving Congress last, fanfared and lauded, feared and accompanied by his new Empress Marie-Louise, come thus far (before being despatched back to Paris!) to show the King of Rome to her Austrian parents and the entire assembled diplomatic throng besides. All will declare it! The destiny of Europe resides in this fated and fêted child of the greatest conqueror to ever have lived. What hocus! The Emperor Napoleon marches on Russia a sick and deluded man. As it has ever been, he searches in conquest for the immortality he'll not find in flesh and blood. The unspoken malady still consumes him. God have mercy on any world that must suffer the ambitions of a man so afflicted.

Crossing Out The Emperor

Michael Black

TELLING STORIES No.1

6 July, in the morning

My angel, my all, my very self -

Only a few words today and at that with pencil (it is yours) - Not till tomorrow will my lodgings be decided - what a waste of precious time - Why this deep sorrow when necessity speaks? - Can our love endure except through sacrifices, through not demanding everything from one another; can you change the fact that you are not wholly mine, I not wholly thine? - Oh God, look out into the beauties of nature and comfort your heart with that which must be - Love demands everything and that very justly - *thus it is to me with you, and to you with me.*

My angel, my all, my very self. A man in love with a woman in all heart and soul and thought and deed! Just like all love should be!

So opens Beethoven's Letter to the Immortal Beloved, but it belongs to all of us really, because everything about loving each other always must. So if you've got the idea into your head that love like this only happens to *artists* or *geniuses* or *great men* then get the same idea back out of your head immediately!

The first biography of Beethoven, published in 1840, assures us that the letter was written in 1806, and is addressed to the Countess Giulietta Guicciardi, then twenty two. "The Countess Giulietta Guicciardi". *Just listen to that name.* With a name like that, you've just got to be staggeringly beautiful, and by all accounts apparently, she was. Giulietta *inspired* Beethoven to write the *Moonlight* Piano Sonata, which just *sings of elegance, beauty and love*! Scholars however have almost totally failed to notice this and this is where the arguments about Beethoven's letter start. For example, Beethoven's first biographer says the Letter to the Immortal Beloved dates from 1806, but the *Moonlight* dedication dates from five years earlier, in 1801.

The Bostonian Alexander Wheelock Thayer, the first reliable 19th century biographer of Beethoven, destroyed the Giulietta Guicciardi case by pointing out that in 1806, the 6th of July did not fall on a Monday, and a later portion of the Letter to the Immortal Beloved is dated "Evening, Monday, July 6". In establishing that the letter could only have been written in 1795, 1801, 1807 or 1812, Thayer appears to have felt very proud of himself, and proposed the recipient as one Therese von Brunsvik.

The evidence that supports this runs as follows. Therese gave Beethoven her portrait in oils, which he retained until his death. Beethoven wrote a letter to Therese's brother Franz that reads "Kiss your sister Therese". Hmm. *That's a bit weak, isn't it?* More convincingly, Beethoven dedicated his Piano Sonata Op.78 to Therese in 1809. And Giulietta Guicciardi (she was still in the plot, but now *the story had changed*) once commented to Otto Jahn "Count von Brunsvik... adored [Beethoven] as did his sisters, Therese and the Countess Deym." Or at least, that's Otto Jahn's story.

This evidence is plausible, but it's still *pretty thin*. And besides, Thayer casts dark shadows of doubt all over his own case by still insisting that the letter was written in 1806. What?! *But Thayer's the one who established that in 1806; the 6th of July did not fall on a Monday!* Yes, that's right. But Thayer also concluded that Beethoven got the date wrong. Another American, Maynard Solomon, a prominent modern scholar of Beethoven, delights in his destructions by pointing out this total brain storm in Thayer's thinking, but Maynard

Solomon has his own candidate to argue for, as we shall see. Thayer's conclusion that Beethoven got the date wrong, although totally speculative, nevertheless strikes me as reasonable. Beethoven frequently got his age wrong in Heaven's name! And surely, anyone who regularly gets their age wrong can get the day or the date of the year wrong easily. Maybe Beethoven didn't think your age had much to do with being in love! But that's a speculation all of my own.

Back to scholastic reality. If, in defence of Thayer, we accept that Beethoven getting the date wrong is plausible, we must also accept that the date of the letter *could be* 1806, in which case, the Countess Giulietta Guicciardi must surely come back into the picture. In other words, whether Beethoven got the date wrong or not, Thayer is contradicting himself after all, though not for the reasons advanced by Maynard Solomon!

Let's forget about the scholastic evidence altogether. The French film maker Abel Gance made a film about Beethoven's Letter to the Immortal Beloved. It's called *Un Grand Amour de Beethoven*. Like anyone with a decent imagination, Gance leaves the scholarship in the library where it belongs, and comes up with the following plot containing pieces of everything:

The Immortal Beloved is Giulietta Guicciardi. Beethoven meets Giulietta in the Salons of Vienna in 1801. He loves her, but she feels only great friendship and admiration for him. One summer night, as Beethoven is improvising the piano piece that becomes the Moonlight Sonata, Giulietta confesses to Beethoven that she is about to marry the young and handsome Count Wenzel Robert Gallenberg. Beethoven tries to dissuade her. Giulietta's mind is made up. Deeply wounded, Beethoven flees outside into a raging storm.

He stays out all night, seeking sanctuary at the old windmill in the village of Heiligenstadt. Some time later, Beethoven returns to Vienna and shuts himself off. The one person to whom he will open his door is the sweet, selfless, loving Therese von Brunsvik, who is also Giulietta's cousin. An old friend, Therese has correctly guessed the story behind Beethoven's broken heart. Beethoven confides in her. At Giulietta's wedding, Beethoven angrily pounds out a funeral march on the organ, greatly upsetting the ceremony. Events prove Beethoven's prescience. After the wedding, Count Gallenberg quickly shows himself up for a gambler and a cad. Giulietta, despairing herself, comes to understand Beethoven's despair. But Beethoven has by this time grown so used to confiding his misery in Therese that the two have grown closer than Giulietta has realised. Unsure of herself, but knowing of no other course, Giulietta, deeply unhappy, confesses her marital error anyway and asks Beethoven to forgive her. Beethoven thinks it's all come rather late, and Giulietta leaves, the two still unreconciled. But reflecting alone, Beethoven is overcome by Giulietta's honesty, and sits down to write the Letter to the Immortal Beloved. At this point, Therese arrives, finds the letter and thinks it is meant for her. Beethoven dares not tell her the truth. In so lying, Beethoven spares Therese her feelings, but ruins his own hopes of happiness. And, by inference, those of Giulietta.

I like this story. It has most of the ingredients such stories need. It has an unhappy marriage, it has raging storms. In the *Moonlight* episode, it connects romantic love and artistic inspiration. In the funeral march episode, it has the romantic foreshadowing of doom, an essential element in all tales of unhappy love. It also has two different cases of irreconcilable unrequitedness. Beethoven and Therese share each other's predicament, but cannot share a union. And it has torn obligations and incestuousness aplenty. Everyone in the story knows everyone else very well. By the end, everyone also knows they can never be happy in love. Beethoven can't hurt Therese, and in all probability, neither can Giulietta. Ironically, Therese is probably the least unhappy. She finds a limited happiness in mistakenly believing that Beethoven loves her, even if he doesn't. Whereas Giulietta and Beethoven, who do love each other, can never consummate their passion. In Gance's film, Giulietta is much prettier than Therese (in real life, Therese had a slight curvature of the spine). It's probably the case that Therese, inexperienced, has had a crush on Count Gallenberg. It's probably the case that Giulietta has always inadvertently lured the men Therese fell for towards her instead. This is ultimately the reason Giulietta cannot push Therese out of the way. It's happened too many times before. And then more irony. Therese wants to be attractive to men as Giulietta is attractive to men, but what Therese wants only makes Giulietta miserable. Therese finds more happiness than Giulietta without Giulietta's looks.

Another thing this story doesn't have is any foundation in fact. Does this matter? *Imaginatively*, of course not. *Evidentially*, yes, at which point we meet the scholars, ever more fusty, once again. If we are to concentrate on Giulietta Guicciardi and Therese von Brunsvik, we get stuck on 1806 again, regardless of the date or day of the week. Because Gance sets his story in 1801. And besides, Giulietta Guicciardi didn't marry Count Gallenberg until 1803, at which point she and her husband left to set up home in Naples. At this point we realise that all our previous concentrations on 1806 count for nothing. Giulietta wasn't around in 1806. *Of course she wasn't around!* That's why Beethoven was sending her a letter! Yes, but the letter states "We shall surely see each other soon" which is extremely unlikely if Beethoven was in Vienna and Giulietta was in Naples. And Beethoven states that he's writing *his* letter with *her* pencil. *So, Giulietta was sending Beethoven pencils from Italy, was she?* And besides, later on, the letter states Beethoven intends to send it to somewhere entitled only "K." And Naples starts with an N. In fact, 1806 has been foisted on us throughout by the complete unreliability of the first Beethoven biography. 1806 is a red herring.

So let's leave Giulietta and ask a new question. *Who are the other candidates for the Immortal Beloved?* The full list runs something as follows; Giulietta Guicciardi, Therese von Brunsvik, Josephine Deym, *née* von Brunsvik, who was Therese's sister. There is also Therese Malfatti, but Thayer's biography argues against her (she just shared a christian name with the first von Brunsvik sister, and was the niece of one of Beethoven's doctors). And then there is Dorothea von Ertmann, the singer Magdalena Willmann, the virtuoso pianist Marie Bigot, the Countess Marie Erdödy, the Berlin singer Amalie Sebald, the poetesses Rahel Levin and Elise von der Recke, the Princess Marie Leichtenstein (once described as "Vienna's most beautiful woman") Marie Pachler-Koschak, the actress Antonie Adamberger, the writer and amateur painter Bettina Brentano von Arnim, and Antonie Brentano, who was Bettina's sister-in-law. Goodness gracious! What a list of fusty endeavour! How about that for the efforts of over a century's scholastic minds! There's an academic industry here. How do we pick our way through it?

Let's start with what we know for sure. Most of these women were well known Viennese beauties. And Beethoven knew most of them through his piano playing. He either taught most of these women the piano, or, having met them socially, subsequently dedicated a piece of piano music to them, however minor. Most of these women were around ten years younger than Beethoven, and we know younger women frequently took his eye. In the caste bound atmosphere of Habsburg Vienna, most of these women were considered socially *superior* to Beethoven, whose initial position as a piano teacher gave him a status somewhere *above* tradesman but *below* court artist.

But what about the women? Forget about Beethoven's letter for a minute, and let's look for a letter going the other way. Let's look for a letter going from one of these women to Beethoven. Unfortunately, there aren't many of these that have survived. But there is one, written by Josephine Deym, which at least acknowledges that there was *something* between them. Some of the evidence in Josephine's favour as the Immortal Beloved is the same as that for her sister Therese. *"Count von Brunsvik adored [Beethoven] as did his sisters, Therese and the Countess Deym."* And there is supporting evidence that Josephine's marriage to Count Deym, by whom she had four children, was deeply unhappy. The marriage was forced on Josephine by her father, and Count Deym was thirty years her elder. But it is Josephine's letter that lifts her up for serious consideration. In 1805, she wrote to Beethoven:

> An inexpressible feeling that lies at the bottom of my soul has made me love you. Before I knew you, your music carried me away with enthusiasm for you. Your goodness of character and your fondness for me have done the rest. The favour you have accorded me, the pleasure of your visits would have been the most beautiful jewel of my life, if only you loved me in a less physical manner. Do not berate me if I cannot respond to this physical love. I would have to break sacred bonds were I to follow your entreaties. Please believe me that I suffer the more in fulfilling my duties and that my actions are certainly guided by noble intentions.

So, the love between Beethoven and Josephine was mutual, but then there were problems. Beethoven wanted to sleep with Josephine. But Josephine was unable to respond. Consider the drawing room scene this conjures up:

Beethoven arrives at the Deym Palace to hear Josephine's piano exercises. Josephine is excited to see him, but also apprehensive after Beethoven's intimations the last time. She also knows that Beethoven cannot for the life of him understand why she is married to the shrivelled up old Count. Josephine is nervous, and plays her exercises badly, conscious throughout of Beethoven's proximity at her side. Beethoven chastises her for not practising. Josephine assures him she has been. Beethoven asks her what the matter is. Josephine moves away to the window. After a silence, she asks Beethoven to play the piano. Beethoven, whose patience with social nicety never lasted long, finds courage in the fact that Josephine isn't looking at him. He proceeds to tell her exactly what he wants to do, and suggests they do it over the piano. Josephine turns around abashed. The passion that she loves in Beethoven's music terrifies her when it is unabstracted and stands before her as flesh and pulsing blood. But Beethoven persists. If not here and now, then how about a secret rendezvous? Josephine is appalled, not only at the suggestion, but also at the secret excitement it causes within her. This is not only because Josephine Deym is married. In fact, she knows full well that the Count will be dead within the year. It is also because, knowing of his own decrepitude, the dying Count has made Josephine take religious vows of chastity. What is Josephine to do?

I like this story. I like it because it is open about sexuality - well, almost. This gives it a certain honesty. It is possible, is it not, that Josephine's letter is a reply to Beethoven's Letter to the Immortal Beloved, refusing him in the kindest possible way once again. In which case, Beethoven's letter dates from 1805 (we do get stuck again here on the date of Beethoven's letter being wrong, but we've discussed that one already.) This suggestion is totally speculative, but at least it establishes a hypothetical dialogue between two lovers. And a great many fusty researches into the Immortal Beloved fall down at this point. They forget that where there is one letter, there is generally another, largely because the scholars are much more interested in Beethoven than they are in the women they are speculating about. It is probably no coincidence that all but one of the fusty scholars I speak of are men.

But let us believe in the Josephine Deym story for at least one glimpsing moment, and accept that the Letter to the Immortal Beloved dates from 1805. Then it follows on that the consuming passion between Beethoven and Josephine must have remained unconsummated for another seven years. And then Josephine's chains of chastity, so troublesome to her in 1805, were briefly released. The really truthful, but totally and utterly unsubstantiated evidence about Josephine Deym and Beethoven dates from 1812. According to Sigmund Kaznelson, what happened goes something like this:

In 1810, Josephine Deym, lonely and unfulfilled by her work for the church, remarries, to one Baron Christoph von Stackelberg. But this marriage, like her first one, soon proves unhappy. Von Stackelberg finds her unwilling to conjugal demands. Josephine, still feeling subject to vows of chastity Count Deym forced her into, feels unable to freely give herself. Von Stackelberg drinks, slaps Josephine around and takes to prostitutes. And then, the final ignominy. In 1812, Count von Stackelberg abandons her, spreading rumours Josephine is frigid. Josephine seeks out Beethoven, and hearing he is at Teplitz, takes flight from Vienna. In Teplitz, she finds Beethoven's lodgings by asking the postmaster. As Beethoven opens the door, for the first time in her adult life Josephine Deym knows exactly what she must do. And she does it. She closes her eyes and gives herself, utterly, totally and completely. This time, it is Beethoven who is overwhelmed by another's passion. Josephine Deym opens her eyes, and finds she can see straight at last. And then she feels ashamed. Again. Exactly nine months later, Josephine gives birth to a little girl, soon christened Minona.

Hhhhhmmmmm. I like this story. I like it because it relieves a very tortured and unhappy woman of the burden of vows she could not keep. And I like it because it provides Beethoven with the child he never had. But there as so often before, an otherwise good story breaks down. Evidentially, it's simply too speculative. If Josephine rendezvous-ed with Beethoven at Teplitz, then why are there no records of her being there? *Well, because Josephine was still a married woman, and she chose to travel incognito. Don't you see, that's also the reason the letter is to Beethoven's "Immortal Beloved!" It was too risky to write down Josephine's name.* Well, no, I don't see actually, because if the story's true, then how come Beethoven took no particular interest in Josephine's little girl? *Beethoven loved children.* Well, maybe Josephine didn't tell him. *But why not?* And it's even more unlikely she wouldn't have told her sister Therese. The two were very close, and Therese had first hand experience of the agonies Josephine went through. Whilst Josephine was married to von Stackelberg, Therese was governess to her children! If anything like this had really happened between *Pepi* and *Luigi*, as Josephine and Beethoven frequently called each other, Josephine would definitely have told

Therese! And in all of Therese's voluminous Diaries, there is not the slightest hint that Josephine's youngest child was Beethoven's.

As ever, we find ourselves in the situation where solving one problem creates another one. For example, if Beethoven wrote the Letter to the Immortal Beloved in 1811 (the earliest date he is known to have been in Teplitz), then Josephine's letter of 1805 can't have been a reply to it. *But there was a real ever-broken love story between Josephine Deym and Beethoven!* Years later, on the 4th February 1846, Therese von Brunsvik wrote in her Diaries:

Beethoven! It is like a dream that he was the friend, the confidant of our house - a magnificent spirit! Why didn't my sister J take him as her husband when she was the widow Deym? She would have been happier with him than with S.

Ultimately, this says it all. *There's not a story ever dreamt of that can save Josephine.* Whatever her traumas with von Stackelberg, she was doomed from her marriage to Count Deym onwards. After the death of the Count, Josephine's other sister, Charlotte, writes to Therese of Josephine's "dreadful nervous breakdown. Sometimes she laughs, sometimes she weeps, after which comes utter fatigue and exhaustion." Josephine rouged her lips; she made up her face, both to an obsessive degree. Josephine Deym was not a happy woman, and that's that. She was to die in 1821 aged a mere forty two, her nerves shot to pieces. Therese, however, whilst never marrying, lived on until the ripe old age of 86, finding consolation by working with homeless children and organising schools for orphans. She lived long enough to read the first biography of Beethoven when it appeared in 1840. Therese was no fool. Reading of the first investigation into the identity of the Immortal Beloved, Therese notes:

November 12, 1840. ... Letters of Beethoven's purported to be to Giulietta. Could they be a fraud?

So, Therese knew it wasn't Giulietta all along!

Who else shall we investigate? I'm not going to advance Bettina Brentano von Arnim's case. Bettina is very good at talking for herself:

When I saw him of whom I shall now speak... I forgot the whole world - as the world still vanishes when memory recalls the scene - yes, it vanishes... It is Beethoven of whom I now wish to tell you... I am still not of age, it is true, but I am not mistaken when I say - what no one, perhaps, now understands and believes - he stalks far ahead of the culture of mankind. Shall we ever overtake him? - I doubt it, but grant that he may live until the mighty and exalted enigma lying in his soul is fully developed, may reach its loftiest goal, then surely he will place the key to his heavenly knowledge in our hands so that we may be advanced another step towards true happiness.

This is gushy and hifalutin to say the least, but also extremely enthusiastic. It's safe to say that Bettina, "still not of age" was more than a little infatuated. She goes on:

[Beethoven] himself said: "When I open my eyes I must sigh, for what I see is contrary to my religion, and I must despise the world which does not know that music is a higher revelation than all wisdom and philosophy..."

All this Beethoven said to me the first time I saw him; a feeling of reverential awe came over me... I was surprised too, for I had been told that he was unsociable and would converse with nobody. They were afraid to take me to him; I had to hunt him up alone... I found him in the third story [of his lodgings and] walked in unannounced. He was seated at the pianoforte.

As you can see, Bettina was more than a bit pushy; she was full of herself too. Later,

[Beethoven] accompanied me home and on the way he said many beautiful things about art, speaking so loud and stopping in the street that it took great courage to listen to him. He spoke with great earnestness and much too surprisingly not to make me forget the street. [My family] were greatly surprised to see him enter a large dinner party at home with me.

Elsewhere, Bettina describes walking "hand in hand with Beethoven". A romantic coup for a young girl indeed.

But what effect did this initial meeting with Bettina have on Beethoven? It had the following:

Vienna, August 11, 1810
Dearest Bettine:

No lovelier spring than this, that I say and feel it, too, because I have made your acquaintance. You must have seen for yourself that in society I am like a frog on the sand which flounders about and cannot get away until some benevolent Galatea puts him in the mighty sea again. I was really high and dry, dearest Bettine; I was surprised by you at a moment when ill-humour had complete control of me, but in truth it vanished at sight of you, and I quickly threw it off. I knew at once that you belonged to another world than this absurd one to which with the best of wills one cannot open his ears... Dearest Bettine, dear girl!... How dear to me are the few days in which we chatted...

Here we have it, a burgeoning romance! Note how, as in all such romantic documents, the arrival of love brings Spring in its metaphoric wake, despite the fact it's actually late summer. I suppose if a man can get the day and date of the week wrong, he's allowed to get the season wrong if he's swooning. Beethoven's noble spirit (so beyond the comprehensions of mere mortals like you and me!) has found its spiritual maiden at last! And, still young herself, there's no curvature of the spine, no chains of chastity or unhappy marriages to overcome here. *Hurray for Bettina!* Surely that's the meaning of Beethoven's letter, save to add Beethoven knew nothing about frogs (there's not a sea-living frog on the planet. Frogs live in ponds and lakes, and just *love fresh water*). *Bettina's our girl!* It remains for me now to simply run the rest of the Letter to the Immortal Beloved, and construct a scenario which explains a rendezvous between our two star-crossed lovers in all its *secretiveness*, perhaps because Bettina's parents didn't approve, for example.

But there's just one problem. Beethoven never wrote the above letter in the first place. Bettina in fact wrote it for him, and published it, along with her other "correspondence" with Beethoven in 1839. *What an audacious fraud!* The rouse was discovered when Otto

Jahn interviewed Bettina about these letters some time later. She immediately became "visibly embarrassed" and could produce no originals. This is disappointing so far as the identity of the Immortal Beloved is concerned, but at least Beethoven stands zoologically excused. Beethoven knew nothing about frogs, but then he didn't pretend to. Bettina's the one with the frog problem, with or without the added Classical allusions. By casting herself as Galatea (a statue of a maiden Aphrodite brought to life for the sculptor Pygmalion, whom had fallen in love with his own creation), Bettina presumably saw herself as both a reflection of and inspiration for Beethoven's art. Or, returning once again to the frog, perhaps Bettina saw herself as the Princess in the fairy tale who kisses her Prince to free him from the curse of frog-dom that the wicked witch had imposed on him so many years before (this would be Bettina's ultimate intention. In the letter, she's still at the point where she's simply keeping her frog-Prince alive, although putting a frog back in salt water would actually *kill any such creature immediately* from dehydration.) Either way, we really should have known all along the letter wasn't genuine, and Bettina's account of meeting Beethoven must be considered rather suspect too. The mature Beethoven, although reasonably well versed in Greek mythology and in fairy tales, seldom refers to either in his letters or in his music.

It's not so much that Bettina was an out and out liar; it's more that she's telling very big fibs in this particular regard. Variously poet, essayist and short story writer, an amateur painter as well as being musical and fluent in several languages, there was not a lot Bettina Brentano didn't think she could do. And, to be fair, one thing Bettina could do it seems, was make Beethoven change his coat, however briefly. Beethoven, in today's parlance, was a *grunge* dresser. He dressed down to the extent that he wasn't bothered about what he was dressed in at all. This leads us to the following short story:

Infatuated and awe struck after her first meeting, Bettina Brentano invites the great Beethoven, so far in advance of the culture of humankind, to dinner at her brother Franz's. Beethoven, as ever bent over his piano, absent mindedly agrees.

That's a *short* story if ever there was one. Now for the sequel:

Despite Bettina's constant attempts to sit closer by Beethoven at the piano stool, and despite her suggestion that the two of them play four hands, the great Beethoven eventually shows Bettina to his door. He stands there unshaven, head of hair standing on uneven ends, his torn shirt missing buttons, and holes in his shoes. Bettina looks him up and down from head to toe, knowing her brother Franz's will be having a very posh do indeed. She can't tell Beethoven he needs to overhaul his entire appearance, so she limits herself to the suggestion he buy a new coat. "Oh" replies Beethoven, "I have several good coats" and beckons Bettina back into his lodgings. "Is that your bed?" inquires Bettina, never one to risk an innuendo being too subtle, but Beethoven is oblivious. "Look!" he says, before opening his wardrobe to reveal a whole array of coats. Bettina goes through the wardrobe as Beethoven proudly eyes his collection. All the coats are shabby, but, sighs Bettina, they are at least less shabby than the one he normally wears, which hangs raggedly by the door. The one Beethoven normally wears is the oldest. "Which one do you think I should put on?" Beethoven changes into the coat Bettina thinks he looks smartest in, and off out into the street they go. Bettina has just succeeded in making Beethoven take her hand in his, when Beethoven insists on returning to his lodgings. He says he doesn't feel comfortable, and wants to put his oldest coat back on again. He says he doesn't feel happy in anything else. Bettina, keen to be with the great man whatever he's wearing (or isn't), acquiesces, and the two of them go off to brother Franz's for dinner, Beethoven looking as much like a tramp as usual.

I like this story. I like it because I think it's amusing. And I like it because whatever the *notorious* unreliability of any account by Bettina, it also has a ring or two of truth about it. And, if it's true, perhaps Bettina did have an altogether remarkable effect on Beethoven after all. Maybe she even persuaded Beethoven to buy a new coat, never mind change one! Because in 1810, the same year that Bettina speaks of first meeting him, something very odd happened to Beethoven indeed. *He started paying attention to what he was wearing.* Everyone around him commented on the change. This story goes something as follows:

In 1810, Beethoven returned from having dinner at Bettina's brother Franz's. It was a very posh do indeed, and Beethoven, suddenly socialised by romance, realises he looks like a tramp. "I look like a tramp" he says to himself. At the dinner party, he had felt thoroughly awkward throughout, and now, in love with his own brought to life Galatea, he decides to do something about it. For the first time in his life, Ludwig van Beethoven becomes concerned about his personal appearance! "I look like a tramp" he keeps repeating in the mirror, pausing only to notice the mirror is broken. And so he borrows a mirror from his friend Zmeskall, and, handing over some money, asks Zmeskall to buy him another one at the same time. Beethoven decides to transform himself. He still loathes shopping, and so he sends another friend, Gleichenstein, a considerable sum with which to buy fine quality Bengal cotton shirts and "at least half a dozen neckcloths." And loathsome of shopping or not, Beethoven himself pays a visit to Joseph Lind, the finest tailor in Vienna, and orders both a new suit and a new coat! Oddest of all, and by now Beethoven is feeling very odd indeed, he writes to his "old friend" Wegeler, and, after apologising for not having written in the previous nine years, asks Wegeler to secure a copy of his certificate of baptism, and to take great care he secures the right one, for there was another Beethoven born and christened Ludwig before him. As Beethoven, donning his new coat, puts the letter in the posting box, he remarks to himself how fortunate it is that Wegeler is now a doctor in Bonn, Beethoven's very birthplace. Wegeler receives the letter and concludes there is only one possible explanation. Astounded by the new sartorial king of musical composition, a great many Viennese, from shoe shiner to tailor to the Immortal Beloved herself, conclude there is only one possible explanation too. Ludwig van Beethoven intends to be married! As all and sundry come to congratulate Beethoven on how well he's looking, only one question remains. Who is he getting married to?

I like this story. I like it because it contains a transformation, a kind of frog-to-Prince piece of magic all of its own. Made up letters or not, perhaps Bettina had the rapturous effect on Beethoven that he'd obviously had on her after all. Perhaps Bettina's still the Immortal Beloved despite her own dishonest efforts that have disqualified her so far. *Well no, I'm afraid not.* Because if Beethoven started to dress properly in 1810, it's safe to say Bettina had nothing to do with the reason why. Because in 1811 Bettina Brentano married the poet Achim von Arnim, by all accounts, the marriage proved a long and very happy one. Further, upon hearing of the marriage, Beethoven sent Bettina a very lame sonnet he'd composed himself for the occasion, which hardly suggests the marriage had broken his heart. So, if Beethoven was planning on getting married in 1810, the question still hangs there unanswered and seemingly unanswerable. *Just who was he planning on getting married to?* George Marek suggests he was planning to marry Therese Malfatti, but the evidence is all but invisible as far as I can see, and besides, Thayer had already pointed out that Therese Malfatti can't be the Immortal Beloved in his much earlier biography. It seems much more likely that Beethoven was preparing to marry Josephine Deym. We know her sister Therese at least retrospectively thought it a good idea and Josephine did marry in 1810, albeit disastrously to von Stackelberg. Maybe she only married von Stackelberg because she, or Beethoven, changed their minds at the last moment. But there's no evidence either way. And so Beethoven's very strange and sudden flirtation with sartorial elegance in 1810 must remain tantalisingly unexplained. And besides, if Beethoven got the date of the Letter to the Immortal Beloved right, then 1810 doesn't fit in, lying awkwardly between the acceptable dates of 1807 and 1812. And if Beethoven didn't get the date right, then we still have no real candidate for the Immortal Beloved in 1810 anyway. No matter how hard we try to make Bettina Brentano fit the evidence, she keeps *proving she's not the one we're looking for*. She made up letters Beethoven was supposed to have sent her, and she married someone else the following year anyway. So how do we explain Bettina's inventions?

Bettina was brought up in a convent, where she quickly astounded the nuns not only by her quickness of mind but also by her excessive vanity. She read avidly in many languages. Her heroine was Helen of Troy, the face that launched a thousand ships, and she fancied herself as a Heloise in search of an Abelard (though preferably not castrated). She studied all she considered to be "beautiful and spiritual", and could quote romantic poetry by the yard. Above all, the young

Bettina Brentano had style. As a teenager, she loved to pose in the convent gardens beneath a Weeping Willow tree and next to a trickling stream, forlorn and pale and wan. As far as Bettina was concerned, there was only just enough water flowing to keep her alive. She was a princess locked up in a tower. As far as Bettina was concerned, there were only two things the convent lacked. One was a mirror, and the other one was men. Bettina early determined to be somebody, but in a society so lacking in opportunities for women, this proved difficult to achieve in its own right. And so Bettina Brentano early took to seeing herself as the Muse for a Great Man.

I like this story. I like it because it sympathises with constriction without taking the subject's frustrations too seriously. Bettina as *Muse for a Great Man* is of course where Beethoven comes in and also where Johann Wolfgang von Goethe, Germany's most famous poet, comes in too. Bettina managed to inveigle herself with Goethe far more than with the Ludwig you are hopefully growing to love. In 1832, Bettina published her *Goethe's Correspondence with a Child*, and the child was she. Whilst a great deal of this correspondence is as fictitious as Beethoven's letter Bettina made up for herself, it is beyond doubt that Bettina grew to know Goethe very well. Apparently, when Goethe walked into a room, all conversation ceased. He was always impeccably dressed; he walked with a purposeful and elegant gait. He was the most famous son of Weimar, and famously irresistible to women, most of whom however could only gaze from afar. But not Bettina.

Bettina Brentano soon learnt to play the Muse for a Great Man to perfection. She would sit wrapped in Goethe's cloak whilst looking up at him with her piercing black eyes. In Goethe's head of full-grey hair Bettina saw wisdom and sagacity. In his proud and unbowed back she saw worldly strength and resolution. As Goethe recited his poetry, Bettina's sensuous bosom would rise and fall rhythmically. Bettina, blushing, admitted she wrote poetry herself. Would the Great Man like to read it? The poem Goethe read was a poem written by a woman about sitting at the feet of a Great Man and acting his Muse. Bettina Brentano knew exactly what she was doing. And she knew also that her mother, Maximiliane Laroche, whom she much resembled, had been a lover of Goethe in her own youth. Like mother like daughter. Bettina came to have such an effect on the sixty year old Goethe that she and Goethe's wife Christiane came literally to blows. Christiane had seen off the mother as a rival and she wasn't going to lose out to the daughter at this late stage...

I like this story. I like it because it encapsulates Goethe's vanity, Bettina's beguiling charm, and Christiane's perfectly predictable and righteous fury. *And I like it because it is true.* Two things can be safely said about Bettina Brentano. She wasn't the Immortal Beloved, but she sure was some girl! And it is definitely through Bettina Brentano von Arnim that Beethoven and Goethe came to meet one another.

Crossing Out The Emperor

BURNING BRIDGES

On the 14th of September 1812, Napoleon Bonaparte, the Emperor of the French, ordered his retinue to cease their line of advance, and disembarking from his carriage, proceeded to climb to the very top of the Mount of Salutation, a place where travellers of all nations traditionally kneel and pray upon their first sight of the view beyond. Napoleon felt no need of prayer, but the view still impressed him greatly. Here he now stood at the height of his fame and ambition, at the watershed of his success, a full 1,800 miles from Paris, further than any conquest, even that of Egypt, had taken him before. The master of Europe from East to West, what a legacy of Empire would his young son the King of Rome grow to inherit! Within the luggage of his retinue were carried maps of Turkey and India, for all seemed possible to the great conqueror come so far. On this warm late summer day, the Emperor of the French stood fully the master of all the vastness he surveyed, and he conjectured, of a great deal beyond. Many capitals had Napoleon seen, but the effect of this one was quite magical, and a cry of happiness escaped him. "Here at last is the Holy City of Moscow" he said, turning to his companion Caulaincourt, his Master of Horse. "It is high time."

The effect on Caulaincourt was no lesser than on his master. For four years Armand de Caulaincourt, the Duke of Vicenza, had served as the French Ambassador to the Tsar's court at St.Petersburg, a city of Frenchified elegance barely one hundred years old, but the view of this ancient capital fully took his breath away. The Byzantine magnificence of the Russian soul seemed to finally reveal itself before him. Glistening in the sun stood proudly the domes of six cathedrals and one thousand five hundred churches of peculiarly mystic aspect and outlandish design. Glittering palaces mingled with distant trees, and the Kremlin, a vast triangular mass of towers resembling at once a palace, a castle and a cathedral all, rose like a citadel out of the general mass of groves and avenues. Clusters of gilded belfries and coloured spiralling domes rose skywards like huge turbans (Napoleon hereafter would forever refer to Moscow churches as "mosques.") The entire effect was gigantic, marvellous, outrageous and fantastical. Caulaincourt at once understood the true reason for the difficulties the campaign had presented thus far. The march on Russia had been a pursuit of the secrets of another world.

Soon, cries of "Moscow! Moscow!" was passing back through regiment, rank and many, many thousands of men. Each and every soldier felt his feet lighten with the joy of rest and the bounty their Emperor had promised them would soon be theirs. How often had this thought alone kept them marching, how often whilst they had buried the dead or nursed their own wounds had the thought of looted riches alone sustained them? "Moscow! Moscow!" It was for this they had watched their own number die of sunstroke and strange fevers, for this had they quenched their thirst for five hundred and fifty arid miles across the Russian plains with cattles' blood and horses' urine for want of unpolluted water. For this had they fought the battles of Vitebsk and Smolensk, and for this had they somehow survived the thirteen hours of hell on earth that was Borodino, a battle without question the bloodiest any could recall or dare to imagine.

Thus it was in jubilant mood that the surviving stalwarts of the Grande Armée marched the final miles to the Gates of Moscow, singing songs of battle and conquest in celebration of their own unsurpassed achievements. Never before or since has the Russian countryside been so filled with the sounds of "Malbrouk va t'en guerre" and the *Marseillaise*. There were many in their number who had served in the armies of Napoleon for full twenty years, many who had fought at Austerlitz and Wagram and Marengo, seen Italy, Egypt and all of Syria, toppled half the crowned heads of Europe and laid siege to Vienna not once but twice. But all considered this the day and scene of their greatest conquest. Napoleon, advancing on the city by the Mojaisk road, approached the Dorogomilov Gate with this singing of the Grande Armée ringing in his ears and fully expecting a delegation of civic leaders to await him. In the highest spirits, he wagered with his marshals as to whether the delegation would merely cower in supplication or with some act of mock independence offer him the keys to the city. Though the marshals laughed, they declined to take up their Emperor's suggestion knowing him of old to be the sourest of losers. It proved a wise decision. The Emperor waited at the Dorogomilov Gate for two hours. There was no delegation to be found. Impatient, Napoleon sent staff to reconnoitre the other gates of the city, but each came back with the same story. There was no delegation anywhere.

Still singing though with voices ever harsher, the Grande Armée grew restless. Each and every soldier dreamed of untold luxuries of multifarious kinds, of beds in palaces and treasure troves to last a lifetime. Each of them was eager to lay claim to their stake, but instead they sat with growing ill humour by the sides of the roads and in adjoining bare and stricken fields. As had been their habit throughout, the retreating Russians had left nothing but ravaged lands and fired storehouses for the French to march on with. The soldiers were expectant of the order of final advance at every moment, but as the minutes became hours, and afternoon faded towards evening and dusk, no order came. Eventually, a single gaunt and haunted figure made his way in greeting beyond the city walls.

Interrogated by Caulaincourt, the news he brought was duly relaid to the Emperor. The fellow was in fact a Frenchman who had languished for many years in a Moscow jail, having renegade and republican views. Rostopchin, the city governor, had that very morning freed him along with all the other criminals, who it was explained now constituted Moscow's only occupants. The governor, having executed a Russian of similar beliefs in front of this terrified Frenchman's eyes, had then turned to him and said "Stranger, you have been imprudent, and yet it is only natural you should desire the coming of your countrymen. Go then, and meet them. Tell them there is but one traitor in Russia, and you have just seen him executed." Rostopchin, so the Frenchman regaled, had then turned his horse and exited the city to the south, following the route of the Russian army under General Kutusov. Moscow had been left deserted.

"The city is ours complete then!" rejoiced Napoleon. The Emperor was eager to take residence in the Kremlin forthwith, but Murat, concerned as ever for his brother-in-law's longevity, insisted on entering the city first with an escort of cavalry for fear of any criminal assassins that might lie in wait. And so it was that Murat advanced cautiously towards the bridge over the River Moskva, and finding it destroyed, forded it to approach the Kremlin walls. He found only a few drunkard men and women firing with wanton aim from the battlements, and these were soon suppressed. The released and frequently deranged criminals of the Frenchman's report alone seemed to walk the streets, but upon investigation, Murat also found many official buildings filled to overflowing with terrified deserters, the injured and the abandoned poor. But of the regular inhabitants of Moscow there was no sign. Each and every one of them had chosen to abandon their homes to inevitable pillage rather than give unwilling hospitality to

Napoleon's army. Murat reflected that this was hardly of consequence, but he remained uneasy. He felt like an actor denied an audience. There was none of the inhabitants' hushed awe that normally accompanied the occupation of a city. There were no false smiles, nor nervousness nor well concealed loathing. There was only the occasional drunken obscenity amidst silence.

Napoleon finally entered Moscow on the afternoon of the following day. He made at once for the Kremlin, entering it via the Trinity Tower, the gateway of one of several bridges that negotiate the surrounding moat. Within these walls, the Emperor had no doubt he occupied the seat of all power. Geography alone dictated so, for the Kremlin rises prominent on a hill above the central bend in the Moskva, and is ringed by a crenellated brick wall perfect for the resistance of prolonged siege. Accompanied by Caulaincourt and the Chief of Staff Berthier, Napoleon took stock of the inner sanctum, of the fortress and the barracks, the arsenal, the Granovitaya Palace and the Cathedral of Assumption, feeling utterly foreign and yet at once totally at home. Here was a collection of buildings to fulfil all a monarch's needs and desires! The means of war, ceremony and religion all combined! Berthier, ever the logistitian, observed what ease of communication such close proximity of facilities must allow. Napoleon, however, upon entering the Granovitaya was disappointed by the sparse furnishings and considered it a miserable dwelling for such a powerful sovereign as the Tsar. "But then, he's not so powerful as he was!" he thought to himself. Caulaincourt ventured that the Tsar concentrated his opulence upon the newer capital of St. Petersburg, but Napoleon dismissed this observation as only Emperor's can. "This is Moscow Caulaincourt. There is no more significant a capital on earth. I walk on the Tsar's very soul." Caulaincourt duly followed Napoleon's footsteps up the marble red staircase, reflecting that as in other matters he travelled with a purpose opposite to the Tsar, who would more normally descend the staircase en route to the great cathedral facing it. But Napoleon, whose interest in matters spiritual was at best pragmatic, reached the staircase's very top without pausing to look around him and then walked quickly through three huge drawing rooms and into the great hall, its vast ceiling supported by a huge central pillar and ornamented by many religious paintings expressing far greater reverence for the next life than for the one Napoleon and his two companions presently occupied. Scornfully moving on, Napoleon noted that the Tsar had even evacuated the curtains and shutters from the state bedroom, and then concluded with pleasure that the evacuation had been done in great haste, for many ornaments and much time honoured armour remained. There was even an old golden throne and an amber toilet seat (both in their differing ways most regal), and many fine clocks on the walls that all told the same, and very correct, time. *Tick, tick, tick.* Noticing a convenient space on the wall, Napoleon immediately hung upon it a picture by the court painter Gérard of the King of Rome. "It has been sent to me by the Empress Marie-Louise", he said turning, "and I trust it will inspire us all." Berthier had no doubts. Caulaincourt said nothing, observing instead much cracking in the plaster from where hung many abandoned chandeliers. The Tsar, he could not help reflecting, clearly valued this place more for its past than for its present importance.

The Emperor so installed in his quarters, the troops marched in at last, at their head the elite Imperial Guard, a body of men in uniforms most resplendent, for Napoleon had spared them from any engagements throughout the campaign. As so often before, Berthier's request to his Emperor that there should be no looting whilst he prepared an inventory of supplies went unheeded. Moscow this day was not ransacked, for the troops well knew they must give some regard to their possible winter quarters, but by nightfall it was much denuded. Greed is contagious, and drink a great stimulus. The infantry wandered through ballrooms and libraries of the like ever forbidden to them in France, helping themselves to a bewildering array of fine furs and portable treasures. The officers commandeered whole cellars of wine and installed themselves in princely apartements. Both officers and infantry saw fit to stable the horses in the churches. That night many thousands of men slept with adequate food in their bellies and with a solid roof over their heads for the first time in many months. Many plans and discussions were had about the further exploration of the contents of Moscow on the morrow, although amongst a significant minority of both officers and men there was a generally unspoken but tangible disappointment that there were no decent women to be found to be raped. Otherwise however, all seemed in order. Nobody cared for the vagabonds and criminals that wandered aimlessly through the streets, and nobody noticed that all the fire-engines were unusable and all the fire-floats had been sunk. Prior to his departure, Rostopchin had done more than release criminals.

Napoleon was awoken at 4 o'clock the following morning by the sound of panic all around him. Moscow was in flames, which, aided by a generous breeze, ravaged the wooden frames of many buildings with wanton adventure. At first the Emperor insisted the fire must be accidental. Even the Russians were incapable of such a sacrifice. But many Russian incendiaries were soon caught with combustibles in hand and immediately shot. Others the French strung up from trees. But the city continued to burn, and when Napoleon climbed to the summit of the great Bell Tower of Ivan the Great to see the extent of the damage for himself, he was shocked at the scale of enflaming carnage. "If we conquer London, we shall not burn it" he was heard to mutter, both enraged and astonished that the Russians could so immolate their own capital. "These Russians are barbarians" he reflected, pausing only to observe how nobly the great Cross astride the Bell Tower might adorn some aspect of Paris. The entire north central and western quarters of the city were ablaze, and the air was thick with burning sparks and embers. A single spark could ignite all the munitions of the Kremlin's arsenal! The stable and the palace roof of the Kremlin were catching fire; one of the bridges across the moat had already collapsed. The Imperial guard were busy dowsing the timbers, but it was to little avail, and it was they, ever loyal and fearing for their Emperor's life, who persuaded Napoleon to leave immediately. Napoleon strode forwards through the flames to the crash of collapsing archways, falling rafters and now near molten iron roofs. The ruins hindering his footsteps, he walked across burning ground, walls of fire to either side of him, the air itself scorching his nostrils and tongue. The heat threatened to burn his eyes, and only with difficulty did he keep them open and alert to danger. At length, half deranged horses were found wandering by the river, and with Caulaincourt the Emperor rode over the Moskva bridge and took again the Mojaisk road. They were heading for the Petrovsky Palace, some six miles distant, and already guarded by the troops of the Empress Josephine's son Eugène.

The fire raged for three days until thwarted by an onslaught of rain. Four fifths of the city was destroyed, though many of the churches, amongst them St. Basil's Cathedral, survived by their isolation from other buildings at the centre of great public squares. Thus the churches had been sought as sanctuary by a great many troops, who abandoned the previous equine occupants to their flame demented fate. Sated and to a large extent drunken at the fire's commencement, discipline in the Grande Armée had fallen apart. The larger buildings were all ransacked for their food supplies. Troops stationed outside the city were more preoccupied with grabbing loot for themselves than with putting out the fire, which in truth had soon become so ferocious as to render all actions against it futile. Furs, silks, silver and jewellery were the principle prizes, but a great many possessions from trunks to carriages were abandoned to the flames when found too heavy to drag away. Together, the fire and the French had extinguished in days the wealth of centuries.

When Napoleon re-entered Moscow on the 18th of September, he found only chaos. Bands of inebriated soldiers roamed the streets in rich oriental clothes, aping Tartars and Cossacks. Sergeant entrepreneurs set up markets in the squares at which valuables changed hands for looted commodities such as sugar, coffee and preserves. Amongst the principle customers were the officers, who saw no shame in bargaining for the loot of their men, and were more appreciative of such stolen properties true worth. Bivouacked soldiers with smoke stained faces lined the streets, cooking horseflesh on fires made of the most slow burning mahogany furniture, eating it off silver plate and reclining thereafter on pavement mounted silk chaise-lounges whilst wrapped in Siberian furs. Berthier was in despair. Everything he had planned for the organisation of garrison supplies would now be impossible. He doubted whether enough buildings stood standing to give shelter to the troops, and it soon became apparent that whatever stores had been left by the Russians were now destroyed. The Grande Armée was rich in jewellery but in short supply of bread and grain, which in the upside down economy that soon developed became worth vastly more than any case of fine liqueurs. Further, the peasants of the surrounding areas either refused to sell grain and hay to the French, or burnt their crops in advance of the asking, and besides, any troops sent out to collect it risked attack from bands of Cossacks, whose movements, subject to no military high command, were impossible to predict. The Moscow all had dreamed of, a safe haven of food and shelter for the winter ahead, was utterly destroyed. In its place, Berthier knew, was only the prospect of shortages of all kinds. Further, there was no realistic prospect of re-supply, for the French bases, at Königsburg, Vilnius and Minsk all stood too far back. The loyal Chief of Staff had lived through many crises, but he could not remove from recollection the heated discussions he had witnessed prior to the Grande Armée advancing from Smolensk. When Smolensk had burned, the Emperor had argued the advantages of Moscow. What would he argue now? Berthier, much chastened, kept these thoughts to himself, and Caulaincourt too remained silent. It took eight times the supplies to feed a horse as to feed a man. From where were these supplies supposed to materialise?

Napoleon however was much pleased to find the portrait of the King of Rome in the Kremlin intact. It still hung between its two companion clocks, the inner rooms of Granovitaya Palace having escaped the fire completely. Even the externals of the building stood largely intact. The wooden frames of the common people suffer far more than the stone edifices of monarchs, and the private thoughts of a Chief of Staff have less bearing on strategy than the dreams of an Emperor. Burned or not, this was still Moscow, and Napoleon turned his attention to securing a cessation of hostilities advantageous to the French by communication with the Tsar Alexander. Alexander, Napoleon felt sure, having been deprived of one capital would be only too willing to sue for peace before the Grande Armée marched on his other one. "With

Moscow burned" said the Emperor, "I argue the advantages of threatening St. Petersburg." On the 20th of September, a letter was thus sent to the Tsar, being transported by the brother of the Russian Minister in Kassel. Napoleon's tone was cordial. He assured his fellow Emperor that it was Rostopchin that had burned the city, and that the French, in the name of all civilised conduct, had done much to limit the damage. He suggested discussion of a compromise peace, and confident of an encouraging reply, turned his attention to matters immediate.

Restoring discipline, Napoleon found occupation in organising daily parades and in the organisation of the outlying monasteries as a defensive ring around the city. But he took Caulaincourt's intermittent warnings of the depths of the Russian winter lightly. Caulaincourt he knew to be a pessimist by nature, and besides, stories of birds freezing to death on the wing seemed scarcely credible to this child of the Corsican sunshine. The weather, Napoleon observed, was "as yet as mild as autumn at Fontainebleau." Caulaincourt's concerns grew daily. When he informed Napoleon the Grande Armée was desperately short of horses, he was ordered to buy 20,000 more. But from where? When told supplies of fodder were running low, he was told to forage for more. But how?

The vengeance of the Cossacks grew daily. Every day they took fifty or one hundred foraging French prisoners, delivering many of these to General Kutusov who, whilst he had abandoned the city, still had his army intact some distance to the south. Many more French prisoners were bought from the Cossacks by the peasants whose hatred of the French found expression in many public and gory executions of their human purchases. One French general sought Kutusov out under a white flag to complain of the cruelty inflicted on "poor men going in search only of a little hay." Murat reinforced this appeal by insisting that if the Cossacks persisted, he would be forced to escort all foraging soldiers with cavalry and artillery. "That is exactly what we wish" came the Russians reply. "Would you deprive us of the pleasure of taking your finest horsemen *comme des poules*?"

Napoleon, frustrated by inactivity, quickly became unpredictable and febrile. He poured over his maps, but the impossibility of joining all the maps of Russia together and viewing them whole upon any table frustrated him greatly. Sullenly, he prolonged the taking of meals through boredom and killed time reading the most disposable of novels. *Tick, tick, tick.* The clocks either side of the King of Rome completed their full circle twice daily, and each day brought fresh repetition of their motion. Here was an unthinking confidence in simple purpose that Napoleon in his darkest moments saw much to envy. *Tick, tick, tick.* Each day he waited more anxiously, and each day no letter from the Tsar arrived. *Tick, tick, tick.* Caulaincourt sought to discuss the re-shoeing and re-clothing of horses and men, but Napoleon showed little interest. His mind resisted full discussion of a winter spent in Moscow, which he still dismissed as an unnecessary contingency. His negotiations with the Tsar would see to that. Nevertheless, when the tales of gruesome and mercenary alliance between the loose-reined Cossacks and enraged peasants were related to him, the Emperor's shock was visible to all. Gradually, the strength and unity of Russian resistance was dawning on even Napoleon, but being more used to imposing the strength of his will upon others, this realisation served only to make the Emperor more isolated.

Ever more impatient, Napoleon suggested to Caulaincourt that he should travel to St. Petersburg under the flag of truce. As former French Ambassador to the Tsar, the Emperor was insistent he was the one who would be most acceptable. Caulaincourt refused the mission. He was certain he would not even be received at the court, and knowing the Tsar well, he was certain no truce was possible whilst Napoleon remained in Moscow. "What do you suggest", came the reply, "if I retreat to Smolensk, it will be a defeat in the eyes of the entire world." Caulaincourt simply observed that since the offer of truce would most certainly be dismissed, it was wiser not be made at all. Undaunted, Napoleon turned to General Lauriston, who had succeeded Caulaincourt as Ambassador. Lauriston, knowing that it would be difficult if not impossible to pass through Russian lines without a *laisser passer*, approached General Kutusov who after much delay greeted him with a feigning courtesy and mock interest in his mission. But he refused Lauriston permission to travel, and demanded Napoleon's second letter of truce be entrusted to one Volkonsky, a member of his own staff. Lauriston thanked Kutusov for his assistance, and Volkonsky thus set off, with a recommendation to the Tsar from his General that the communication he carried be ignored. It was. In desperation, for it was now the second week of October, Napoleon sent Lauriston to Kutusov once again, with a request for "arrangements that might give to the conflict a character consistent with the established rules of warfare." Kutusov concluded that Napoleon was now actively fearful of the starvation of the Grande Armée, and replied only that he had no control over any but those in his direct command. For the Cossacks and peasants he could not vouch. The confidence of the Russian General increased as Napoleon's supplies diminished. As October advanced, the Grande Armée took more and more the part of scavengers, whilst Kutusov's supplies burgeoned with delivery from the Don, the Ukraine and the vast steppes to the east.

The troops of the Grande Armée had awaited the reply of the Tsar with as much eagerness as Napoleon himself. The letters of Napoleon they knew of old to be the prelude to the reliable capitulation of the enemy. But as the warfare by stalemate of the Russians became daily more apparent to them, the troops grew anxious and ill tempered, and, finding their faith in the strategies of Napoleon for the first time waning, took to discussing the situation amongst themselves.

The harlequinade of armed adventure that had marched across Europe during the early months of the summer was by now rudely disabused. The Grande Armée had been cheered as they had marched into Vilnius, for the Lithuanians, like the Poles being unwillingly subject to Russian domination, considered the French their allies. But as they had marched further into Russian lands, the hostility the troops encountered had staggered all. The sullen hatred of the peasants and the constant sorties of the Cossacks had no parallel in any other campaign. The veterans of the Grande Armée were particularly shocked, being more used to considering themselves as liberators, the harbingers of freedom. But whilst the peasants lived in misery and hardship, they yet held the Tsar in mystic devotion, and clearly believed the French to be the anti-Christ. And amidst the still smouldering ruins of Moscow, there was mounting disquiet at the casualties. The Grande Armée had crossed the River Niemen and set foot on the Tsar's territories with 600,000 men, but was now reduced to barely 140,000, the vast majority having succumbed to disease and fatigue. On the march from Vilnius to Vitebsk upwards of 40,000 men had been lost in the heat and dust storms of the vast Russian plain before a single shot was fired in battle. The forced marches of thirty miles a day had stretched the endurance of men and the route of supply lines to the very limit. And there had never been adequate hay for the horses. Summer grass, where it could be found, was no substitute for such hard working beasts, and thousands had died, their stomachs bloated as they ate unripe rye. To many troops, as they sat idle awaiting the Tsar's letter of surrender, the whole great enterprise now seemed in large measure absurd. Not only men, but cattle for milk and beef who had never entertained anything more strenuous than a walk from a farmer's yard to a field, had been expected to traverse immense distances. Many of the veterans, recalling Napoleon's lightening victories of the past, now observed how at Vitebsk and Smolensk and even at Borodino no truly decisive battles had been fought. Though bloodied, the army of Kutusov remained intact, and two other Russian armies under Chichagov and Wittgenstein were known to be assembling to the south and north. "He should seek out the Tsar in war, not write him letters" they said. "He's an Emperor now, not a General" all concluded, pondering how the administration of his vast conquests might possibly conspire against single-mindedness. A few cynics recalled how Napoleon had abandoned the remainder of his troops in Egypt in 1799, and that, frustrated at inaction; in Moscow he might yet do the same. But most still retained the faith to resist such worries. One story from the very start of the campaign, however, gained constant retelling. Whilst he reconnoitred the left bank of the River Niemen for a suitable crossing point, it was said Napoleon's horse had been startled by a hare and so discharged the Emperor to the ground. As the days and weeks went by, so the story gathered around its retelling worse and worse portents. Such were the conversations and concerns of soldiers who's debating of strategy, whilst germane, concealed more immediate perils. "An army marches on its stomach" their Emperor once famously remarked, but it survives encamped by its latrines, and the ruins of Moscow were fast becoming an impure cesspit. Surrounded by stench and consumed with boredom, the troops blamed Berthier for the want of supplies they had half destroyed themselves. Inactivity breeds rancour, and rancour breeds itself. But not even the most sagacious of the troops dared imagine a full winter spent in these conditions.

No diplomacy had ever more angered Napoleon than the Tsar's incommunicado. "Moscow", he came to observe "is not a military position. It is a political predicament." Frustrated beyond measure at full five weeks inactivity, Napoleon called his marshals to the Kremlin. They found the Emperor most excited, his eyes shining as he walked back and forth over the maps of Russia he had now triumphantly pieced together on the floor. "We must march immediately on St. Petersburg" he announced. The marshals were astonished. St. Petersburg lay three hundred and fifty miles to the north, the roads would be barren of provisions, and the journey would be bound to take at least six weeks, demanding its completion after the onset of winter. "This represents a huge difficulty" said Caulaincourt, well knowing he proffered greatly unwelcome advice. "You lack stores, horses for the artillery, transport for the sick and wounded, and clothing for the soldiers. Every man must have a sheepskin, stout fur lined gloves, a cap with ear flaps, warm boot socks, heavy boots to prevent frost bite. You lack all this. Not a single frost-nail has been forged for the horses' hooves. How are you going to draw the guns?" Eugène, Murat, and even Berthier were unanimous that the Grande Armée was in no condition to march anywhere, and besides, they would leave Kutusov with a Russian army gaining strength every day to the south that could easily reoccupy Moscow. The Emperor in seeking to conquer two capitals would succeed only in losing both.

"Then what do you suggest?" said Napoleon, whose own march across the room in two strides from Moscow to St. Petersburg seemed to all present a most theatrical display of wishful thinking. "This country is more vast than anything I had comprehended. Consider this. Most of Russia lies further from Moscow than Moscow lies from Paris. This is a country of many countries. It is so vast that it commences to the east of Poland, and wraps itself half way around the globe, finishing only to the west of the Canadian and American wilderness. When in the east it is day, in the west it is night. It defies me! Even the Tsar has scant control over a great deal of it. How am I supposed to conquer a country that has not yet conquered itself?" The marshals were silent.

"The issue is urgent gentlemen. It is proving most difficult to rule the rest of my dominions from this eastern extremity." For the first time since his Coronation, Napoleon found himself pondering the strength of his hold on Paris. The Imperial government was yet young, and many intriguers remained in the capital to oppose him. "And the French are like woman. One should not be away from them for too long. I still say we should march on St. Petersburg this very day. All we need is a fresh victory." The marshals were again silent, but the looks Napoleon could read on their faces made it clear this was an act of united insubordination. They would refuse to lead their troops.

"What do you suggest?" said the Emperor almost beside himself. "I can advance eastwards into central Russia, but what will that achieve save to stretch the supply lines still more? Or I can withdraw to Smolensk and Vitebsk for the winter to start a fresh campaign in the spring, this time making straight for St. Petersburg through Riga. But in the eyes of the entire world that will look like defeat, and I will not do it. Or I can seek a battle immediately with Kutusov to the south, and then continue to the fruitful regions that lie in the Ukraine. But if I go south, I will only have to march north again, for the Tsar still eludes me." Caulaincourt, who had heard this kind of pondering of strategy many times before, nevertheless found himself astonished. The presumption with which Napoleon included within his own first person the lives and prospects of many thousands of men amazed him, as it did that he had never noticed this trait of his Emperor before. Napoleon, still considering the southern option, paused as he stood on Kiev, and then announced "Alternatively, I can winter in Moscow, and march on St. Petersburg in the spring. My mind is made up. This will be the cause of action. Do what is necessary."

Thus the meeting was concluded. Knowing of Napoleon's famed firmness of mind, all present were relieved and yet somewhat perturbed that their Emperor had capitulated in the face of their silent objections to his original plan. Winter in Moscow was however decided, and so the marshals spread the word throughout the Grande Armée. The troops were dismayed. Winter in Moscow! What a dreadful prospect. It would be hell on earth. But their Emperor was their Emperor, and so they resigned themselves to prolonged acquaintance with starvation and impossible cold. It was thus with unprecedented bewilderment that they learnt almost immediately that Napoleon had changed his mind. The Grande Armée was to withdraw westwards and winter at Smolensk.

Wishing to avoid marching back across the same now ravaged lands over which he had advanced, Napoleon planned first to march south. "March to Kaluga" he cried, "and woe betide anyone who obstructs my passage!" With great haste, the troops assembled their loot and booty, hiding a great deal of it beneath the munitions and provisions. In consequence, a great many wagons were overloaded, making the toil of the already weakened horses even more arduous. The Grande Armée that had marched on Moscow with 600,000 men now consisted of 87,500 infantry, 14,750 cavalry and 533 guns, with a train following it of some forty thousand carriages and wagons. The entire effect was of a shambolic caravan, a wandering nation taking with it the salvaged loot of a devastated city almost in desperation, for in truth this was the only reward for their efforts that the troops could claim. The Emperor himself set the tone, taking with him many treasures of the Kremlin along with the great Cross of the Bell Tower of Ivan the Great, which he intended to mount in Paris over *Les Invalides* as a shining testimony to his greatest act of conquest. Napoleon also saw personally to the portrait of the King of Rome, entrusting it to the care of the Imperial Guard. The result was a huge lumbering procession far removed from the light mobility of the armies with which Napoleon had risen to prominence. There was enough food, Berthier claimed, for twenty days, but horse fodder for less than a week. And of adequate winter clothing there was almost none.

The withdrawal (for none as yet dared call it retreat) commenced on the 19th of October. As Napoleon left the city he had entered thirty five days previously in expectant triumph, he found himself strangely pensive and lack-lustre. And oddly for one who considered his name and every action to be synonymous with the future, the Emperor found himself dwelling on the past. Fouché, formerly the head of the secret police, had, upon hearing of Napoleon's intention to march on Russia, argued strenuously against the project, pointing out that Napoleon was already the master of the greatest Empire ever assembled by any one man. Further, all of history argued the impossibility of establishing absolute monarchy. Napoleon left

Moscow with the words of his own reply ringing in his ears. "I have eight hundred thousand men. To one who has such an army, Europe is an old prostitute who must obey his pleasure. Am I to blame because I have a degree of power that forces me to assume the dictatorship of the world? I must make one nation of all the European states, and Paris shall be the capital of the world." At least, reflected the Emperor, no one could consider Moscow any more the capital of anything. The fire and the Grande Armée had seen to that, and what they had started, Napoleon planned to finish. Prior to his departure, the Kremlin was primed with munitions by the Imperial Guard, and it is said that as the Grande Armée marched from the scene, the resulting explosion could be heard for thirty miles. Such was Napoleon's revenge on the Tsar's refusal to write him letters.

The road to Kaluga held upon its way the key town of Maloyaroslavets. Kutusov, not having intelligence that Napoleon had left Moscow until the 22nd of October, nevertheless managed to secure the town for the Russians under Docturov, driving out Eugène's advance guard from all positions save the strategically vital bridge. As more and more troops of both armies converged on this point, the bridge, though miraculously still standing, changed hands no less than seven times. Eugène in particular welcomed the fight. Here was an opportunity to engage Kutusov's army in full battle, and defeating it, thus escape being plagued by its presence throughout the forthcoming weeks. But communications were poor amidst the slow moving confusion, and Napoleon, who was not informed of the battle until mid-morning, failed to send up adequate reinforcements. The French took the town for the loss of some 4,000 men, but the Russians withdrew about a mile to the south still largely intact. Napoleon slept that night in a squalid weaver's hut, no grander dwellings being available. The mansion at nearby Vinkovo, the residence of the same Rostopchin who had burned Moscow, had been razed to the ground. All that was found was a note saying "I voluntarily set fire to this building, not wishing it to be polluted by your presence." As Caulaincourt improvised a curtain to create for the Emperor some privacy, he could only reflect his master looked weary. The cold resolution of his steel grey eyes seemed but a distant memory. "I beat them every time" came the lament from behind the screen, "but I cannot reach the end."

The road to Kaluga was now blocked. Napoleon, demoralised at the thought that however much he advanced south, Kutusov would simply withdraw further, chose to turn north, taking the Mojaisk road that led to the bloody field of Borodino itself. It was with much disquiet that the further diminished ranks of the Grande Armée turned themselves around, now retreating along the line of their own previous advance, the road littered with bayoneted and diseased corpses, the field's bare earth and ashen cinders. They knew along this road they would find no supplies or provisions, but Napoleon now wished to place as much distance between himself and Kutusov as was possible. Though exhausted, there was much disquiet amongst the troops as they considered such a negative strategy. Never before had they sought to avoid any opposing force, being used to seeking such out and crushing them. There was much concern that Kutusov was now free to join up with the two armies of Chichagov to the southwest and Wittgenstein to the north, and thus united, the Russians would be able to expel the French remains with an overwhelming force. The Grande Armée, which had numbered some 100,000 when leaving Moscow now numbered some 90,000 at most, and well knew of its own peril. A strange nostalgia swelled within the ranks. The young Bonaparte would have seen the importance of Maloyaroslavets in advance, and marched on it with much greater speed and number. The young Bonaparte would have marched on both Moscow and St. Petersburg with lightening force, and, reaching both as early as August, would then have negotiated peace from a position of overwhelming strength.

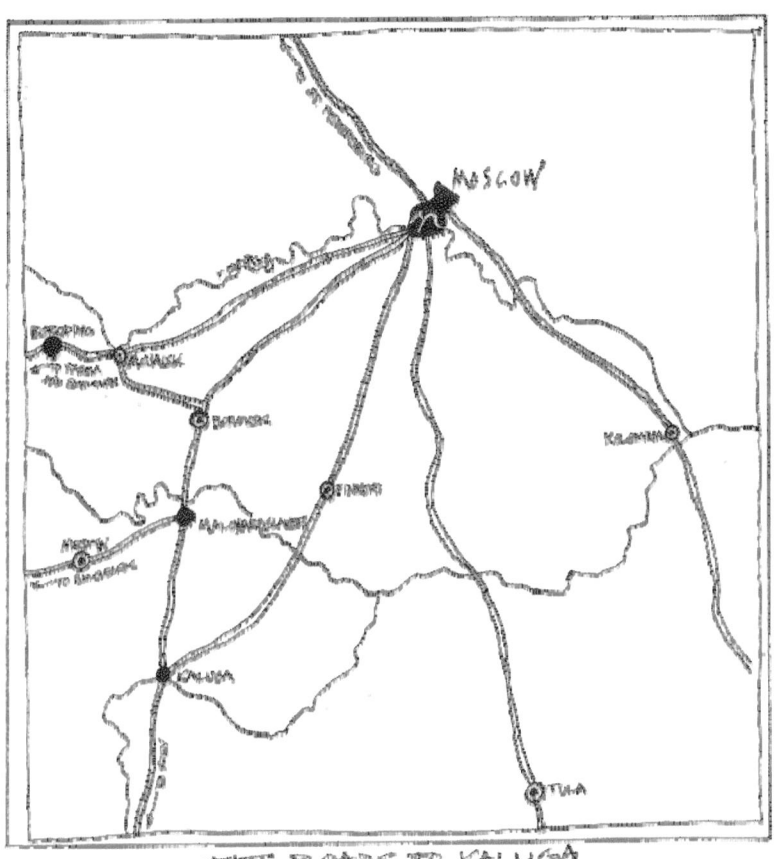

The Emperor himself, who for the most part travelled in his carriage, well warm in his sable cap, fur-lined great coat and boots, heard little of these discontents and speculations. Concerned to make the most of the still clement weather, he ordered the Grande Armée to march some twenty five miles a day, mostly on poor roads and with many soldiers now having only wrapped and oiled rags for footwear. On the 29th of October, they reached Borodino, scene of the battle that had laid open the way to Moscow only seven weeks before. The highway skirts the battlefield proper to the south, and many thousands chose to avert their eyes, the stench from the corpses and the cries of the wheeling carrion crows being sufficient witness to the remnant carnage. But Napoleon stopped his carriage, and rode to the centre of the field. Here, he felt, somehow was the place where his destiny had been decided, though to what end he could not as yet make out. The battered redoubts from where the French and Russians had bombarded one another now resembled extinct volcanoes. Napoleon could still recall vividly the smoke of battle that had consumed them, and yet now they stood silent, all energy spent. All around was the debris of bloody destruction, helmets, swords, bayonets and muskets, broken drums and bloodstained standards. There were dismembered limbs still clutching now ownerless bugles. The wolves and crows had picked the bones of some 40,000 corpses still unburied. What triumph was this? Even here, the one great battle of the campaign, Napoleon had somehow failed to act incisively. He could remember standing here after the battle itself, hearing the Russian camps a thousand yards distant still shouting of their victory. Un-destroyed, they were undefeated. Now on this field of bloodshed he could still see Russian corpses clenching the cross of St. Nicholas, which they had kissed as they lay dying to ease the pain. And he remembered his own illness and how it had dogged him through the battle itself. His maladies had made it impossible to act solely in the interests of glory. He felt constipated; he had difficulty passing water, his hands and feet swelled through constant water retention. He remembered how with relief he had seen the battle not go into a second day, for having lost his voice, he was incapable of command.

Napoleon turned full circle. Almost vomiting at the sight of it, he saw a one legged soldier crawl from the putrid remains of a horse's carcass, his uneven weight supported by a charred plank of wood. Wrapped in a burned and filthy flag of the tricolour, the soldier approached his Emperor, half naked, but wearing a brocaded general's hat.
"What's your name?" said the soldier.
"I am the Emperor Napoleon."
"No you're not. I am."
"I am the only Emperor" asserted Napoleon.
"You're an impostor" insisted the soldier, pulling from his nonexistent scabbard an imaginary sword. "*En garde!*"

Napoleon remounted his horse, ordering that this deranged unfortunate be tended by the medics. "He has lived seven weeks on putrid flesh and stagnant water. I salute him." Napoleon then visited the convent of Kolotskoi, which had been used as the French army hospital during the battle. He found many of the wounded still alive, though many thousands more had perished for want of sufficient cleanliness and surgical equipment. The survivors crawled to the door, extending what supplicating hands they had left to their Emperor. *"Vive l'Empereur! Vive la France!"* they cried. Berthier was instructed to see that as many of these men as possible were loaded onto the carts already over-laden with loot and under-laden with supplies. The Chief of Staff encountered much hostility in carrying out his Emperor's command, and the vast majority of the newly rescued were subsequently dumped by the troops entrusted with their charge. Many hundreds of miles of march remaining, the common soldier could not afford compassion. Napoleon however, left the surrounds of Borodino much heartened by the warmth with which the wounded had greeted him. He took to considering how, resupplied by winter at Smolensk, he would overwhelm St. Petersburg the following spring. That night, the bivouacs of the Grand Armée felt the bite of frost for the first time.

The first flurries of snow fell some six days later. In two days more, it was snowing heavily. The blizzards dictated men marched following only those in front of them, for none could see more than thirty yards. The days grew shorter, and soon it was dark by four o'clock in the afternoon. Men's' breath froze on their beards; their noses turned white and then blue. The rate of progress slowed to some twelve miles, for the army was hindered not only by the weather but also by the treasured loot the troops carried with them, which they were loath to abandon until survival alone dictated it (after all, Napoleon himself still insisted that the great Cross of Ivan was hauled across the ever more frozen terrain.) Stragglers fell exhausted by the road side, awaiting only the snow to cover them in an anonymous grave. The most unfortunate were denied even this, and met instead the revenge of peasants who delighted in beating out their brains. What food was carried in the supply train was reserved for the Imperial Guard, the cavalry, the gun teams and the carriage horses of the officers, whilst the common soldier survived as best he could on pine and willow bark. The horses expired in ever greater numbers to complement the diet of the ranks of the unfortunate, whilst those that survived faired little better. As balls of impacted snow gathered in their hooves, each step became agonising, and on the growing sheets of ice they found it impossible to remain upright. The Grande Armée now resembled a most surprising sartorial procession, wrapped for clothing in the booty of Moscow. It was commonplace to see a soldier, his face dark and repellent, wrapped in a coat of pink or blue satin, trimmed with swan feathers or fox fur. The procession struggled on, wrapped in ladies furs and useless silks, their heads wrapped in a multitude of coloured scarves, their feet frequently protected by nothing more than the same.

The raids of the Cossacks increased daily, but it was the cold that did for most. Amongst the ingenious, it was found that by laying a powder train to a munitions wagon, much havoc could be caused by exploding the wagon's cargo in the faces of the advancing Russians, but this demanded much organisation, and in the main only aggravated Slav revenge. The entire line of march came to resemble an elongated battlefield. In the morning, men would not leave the ashes of the fires they had frequently paid to sit by in spite of the Russians advancing and cannon-balls falling all around them. The extremities of limbs so fast heated by night fires and chilled by the day succumbed with sudden stench to gangrene. Many who swallowed snow to quench their thirst perished as their guts burned in furious reaction. Baron Larrey, the chief surgeon, noted that many of the bald perished first for want of heat retaining hair, but mortality was soon far more widespread. It was common to tell an officer you'd rather die than endure another day of the dreadful march. "The Emperor's losing himself" the infantry cried, "and us with him!" Napoleon now thought only of retreating from the scene with as much haste as possible, and, travelling in the vanguard with the Imperial Guard, showed little interest in the fate of those behind him. Fortune, observed Caulaincourt, had smiled so persistently on him in the past that he seemed unable to face it squarely now it proved fickle.

The Grande Armée that had skirted Borodino with ninety thousand arrived at Viasma with 65,000, only to find the town had already been bombarded by Kutusov. Viasma promised no respite, and indeed consumed energies further. Passing through the town some three days after Napoleon had already left it, the divisions of Murat, Eugène and Marshal Ney found themselves engaged by Miloradovich with a force of 20,000, and lost a further 7,000 men simply in securing the continuance of their line of retreat. By the time the Grande Armée finally reached its planned winter quarters at Smolensk, it numbered only forty thousand. For weeks the men had marched in the hope that here they would find rest, shelter and fresh supplies in abundance. In all three they were disappointed.

General Charpentier, the Governor of Smolensk, had learned of the approach of the Grande Armée only some two days before its arrival, and had no notion of its dilapidated condition. Supplies had steadily been moved in from Germany and Poland, including some cattle on the hoof and many wines and fine cheeses from France. But they were totally insufficient for the purposes required, and by the time the main body of the troops arrived, most of the supplies had already been consumed by the Imperial Guard, who, confident in their status as war veterans, simply ignored the orders Charpentier's administrators had to ration them. But the biggest disaster was the news that on the 16th of November, Chichagov, moving up from Brest-Litovsk, had captured Minsk with its huge supply of stores sufficient for the entire winter, thus rendering any adequate replenishments of Smolensk impossible. Napoleon's admonishment of Charpentier was worse than useless. It was self-deceiving. There was now no possibility the Grande Armée could winter in Smolensk, and a real danger that unless it marched on with the greatest haste it might be captured in entirety, the Emperor amongst it. Chichagov approached from the south west, Kutusov from the east and Wittgenstein from the north, each with the clear intention of capturing Borisov with its bridge straddling the River Beresina. The Beresina, a tributary of the River Dnieper, stood directly across the line of the Grande Armée's retreat, and without the command of the bridge at Borisov, swift withdrawal was not only impossible, but risked the Grande Armée's complete destruction.

The Emperor, whilst privately aware of the ensuing great peril, behaved in Smolensk with a regal insensitivity to the condition of those around him. He asked few questions concerning the wounded, knowing only too well the doctors had inadequate medicines to attend to them. He ignored also the markets the troops set up to sell their loot of Moscow to Smolensk's Russian inhabitants, for most had abandoned all hope of their treasures or themselves surviving all the way to France. Napoleon gave only orders that the towers of fortification that surround Smolensk be blown up, so as not to hinder his progress when next the Grande Armée advanced this way. And then, on the 14th of November, he departed.

Napoleon now commanded the vanguard, and Marshal Ney the rearguard. Between them marched a procession forty miles in length. Newly animated by peril and the possibility of his own personal capture, the Emperor studied his maps with renewed vigour. Nothing, at this advanced stage of withdrawal, was allowed to hinder progress. The Cross of Ivan, which had cost so many lives in hauling it this far, was finally abandoned to the elements, along with the chests that contained the maps of Turkey and India, and many containing gold and silver ingots together with some estimated £200,000 in coin.

Despite these measures, sufficient haste proved impossible in the worsening conditions, and the Grande Armée's progress was now hindered by ever bolder attacks not only of the Cossacks, but from the vanguard of the pursuing Russian armies. Napoleon made the greatest progress, but the rearguard was much delayed. At Krasnoe, Marshal Ney found his way blocked by Miloradovich, and Napoleon, by now some eighty miles ahead, presumed him lost. In fact, Ney conducted a miraculous escape. Napoleon had avoided the perils of crossing the River Dnieper by travelling to its north, but Ney, forced south from Krasnoe, had no choice. Somehow he eluded Russian pursuit and found a bend in the river solid with ice floes, which many soldiers, though no artillery and few horses managed to cross. Napoleon took great heart when he learned of Ney's survival, for he valued him as "the bravest of the brave." But Ney had lost all but 2,000 of the 10,000 in his command, and worse was to follow. When reaching Orsha, Napoleon found only two days supplies and learnt that Chichagov had captured the Borisov bridge two days earlier. Turning to Caulaincourt, the Emperor confided his innermost thoughts. "This", he observed "is beginning to be serious."

News that Chichagov now blocked their exit had a devastating effect on what remained of morale. Even a slight thaw did little to aid men's' spirits, for though it meant they could more easily sleep at night, so they also found marching through mud more laborious than marching over impacted snow. The Grande Armée, though still bearing the name, marched from Orsha to the Beresina with the appearance of a funeral procession, a disorganised mass without shame, many without weapons, its units all mixed in chaos. Officers and men walked side by side with no regard for rank and number. And all marched silent, eyes to the ground like gangs of prisoners, convinced they were marching to their deaths.

The spirits of the Emperor however, excited by the necessity of forging a brilliant strategy of escape, were strangely lifted. "I have played the Emperor for too long" he said. "Now it is time to play the General." His want of troops made certain options impossible. There was no possibility of recapturing the Borisov bridge, and besides, any attempt would risk Chichagov's destruction of it. He could make for the north and by-pass the Beresina entirely, but that risked Wittgenstein reaching the French base at Vilnius before him, and thus would only delay and not evade confrontation. Or he could head south, ford the river at Beresino, and attempt the recapture of Minsk. But the Beresina grew wider as it flowed south, making fording more and more difficult. And besides, he doubted the Russians had left the supplies at Minsk intact.

Napoleon resolved to cross the Beresina as swiftly and as close to Borisov as was possible, thus giving the three still converging Russian armies as little chance of effective pursuit thereafter as could be contrived. His advance parties brought him valuable intelligence of a fording point at Studenka, some seven miles north of Borisov, where, save for a middle section of some twelve feet, the river was no more than three feet deep. But now, the slight thaw that had accompanied the Grande Armée from Orsha became as urgent an impediment as the numbing cold that had preceded it. Every hour at Studenka, the river was rising and the current increasing. Napoleon congratulated himself on not trying to cross further south where the effects of the thaw would be even greater, but the obstacle before him was great enough. The Beresina was soon some twenty feet deep and two hundred feet across. It could not be forded at all, and had to be bridged.

The success of Napoleon's plan depended on convincing Chichagov that he intended to cross the Beresina between Borisov and Beresino, thus luring any Russian troops away from Studenka. And so noisy preparations were made at the three decoys of Ucholodi, Sabashevichy and Borisov itself. Trees were busily felled, sawed and hammered in a simulation of bridge building to deceive Chichagov's spies. At the same time, Napoleon continued to march west direct it seemed to attempt a recapture of Borisov itself, but on the night uniting the 25th and 26th of November he switched north under cover of darkness, arriving at Studenka the next morning, where he rendezvous-ed with General Elbé, his chief engineer.

All the French pontoon bridges had been abandoned without foresight at Orsha, and Elbé was forced to manufacture two bridges from what timbers he could tear from the houses of Studenka and Veselovo. Fortunately, Elbé had salvaged several forges, chests of tools and cart-loads of scrap-iron from the wheels of abandoned carriages, which he used to make crampons to secure the timbers together. Napoleon showed no awareness of how much the success of his plan thus depended on the initiative of another, being too delighted that his own plan of decoy seemed to have fooled the Russians so completely. Some four hundred sappers worked with fury. They built two bridges, each three hundred feet long, one of lighter construction for the infantry and the second for what remained of the cavalry and artillery, this being constructed some two hundred yards down stream. The trestles, twenty three for each bridge, were made after nightfall under the cover of the river bank for fear of the sound of their construction alerting any passing Russian patrol. They were then carried to the river bank and sunk into the bed at increasing depths by men who worked waist and then neck deep in freezing water for hours on end. The deepest central channels were bridged by most comparatively fortunate engineers working from rafts, for few of the almost fully submersed sappers survived. They either died from hypothermia and frost-bite, or found themselves swept down stream by the rising weight of water it was their mission to overcome.

The first infantry of the Grande Armée crossed the foot bridge now secured for them as soon as they reached Studenka, for all knew the deception of the Russians could not last. But there were soon setbacks outside the realm of Russian guns. The artillery bridge quickly buckled, and took several hours to repair. At past midnight of the following day it collapsed again, and whilst what sappers survived re-entered the water to repair it, the now constant arrival of troops, stragglers, artillery and cavalry at the bridgehead only threatened it with complete annihilation. Seeing how tenuous was the artillery bridge, too many attempted to cross the infantry bridge, threatening that with destruction also. There were soon conflicts of priority at every point, and the slow progress across the artillery bridge only reinforced the ever growing crush on its eastern bank. The horses had to be led single file, and the bridge swayed and trembled under the wheels of carriages and the remaining artillery transports.

Total panic ensued when the Russians finally realised Napoleon had tricked them. So long was the train of the Grande Armée that it took a full three days for all to reach the Beresina, and most arrived to find Wittgenstein pounding them with cannons from the east bank whilst Chichagov pounded them from the west. Sappers now worked to keep the artillery bridge from collapse under constant rifle fire. All demarcation of infantry and artillery crossings broke down completely. As more and more of the elite regiments of the Grande Armée crossed the Beresina, so the stragglers still on the eastern side panicked more. With his Imperial Guard across, plus the troops of Ney, Davout and Victor, Napoleon could not risk Russian pursuit across bridges he himself had built.

The Emperor ordered General Elbé set fire to both the bridges at ten o'clock in the morning on the 29th of November 1812. The fires ran quickly from end to end, consuming many then crossing them. The thirty thousand who remained on the eastern shore ran demented in every direction, faced with the bayonets of the Cossacks, the freezing and still rising waters of the Beresina or self-immolation upon the burning and collapsing timbers that now denied them passage. A huge mass of men and horses surged towards both bridgeheads, but the flames threw them back and thus they plunged into the icy river. Exhausted horses were swept immediately downstream, men were cut in two amongst the ice-floes. Some cut their way through the terrified throng with their swords, but, still finding their way blocked upon the banks, fell back to weep in despair. The artillery bridge fell into the Beresina first, and thousands braved the flames of the infantry bridge in a desperate last attempt to escape. But that too collapsed under the sudden weight of desperate humanity it could not support. Many women of the ambulances and canteens braved the ice-floes, many desperately holding on to infants. But these off-spring of the private liaisons of the march on Russia were mostly lost in the deep and treacherous mid-channels of the ever-swelling river, though one it is said survived, its mother managing to cross the Beresina astride a struggling horse, one hand on the bridle and the other pressing her child against her fur wrapped bosom. All hope departed from the despairing multitude who watched this last miraculous escape, and the collective scream of mortal agony became at this moment so universal that it rose shrilly audible over the noise of the elements and the thunders of war and the sustained and redoubled *hourras* of the Cossacks. It haunted many of the survivors of the Grande Armée who now made their way across the Beresina's western marshes. But none dared to look back. All hope was dead.

Napoleon watched this scene with all the calm of a man on parade at the Tuileries. When the thaw came on the eastern banks of the River Beresina in the spring of 1813, still lying there were the bodies of twenty thousand French men and women who had been frozen solid all winter, but the Emperor considered his escape across the Beresina to be one of his finest manoeuvres. "It is my name alone that has protected the army" he reflected. "Here is a triumph to balance the disappointments of the campaign." Now he travelled with increased haste towards Vilnius, a self-appointed "Sacred Squadron" of surviving cavalry protecting his flanks. But upon reaching Smorgoni, he learnt of fresh travails confirming his worries he had been too long absent from Paris. A plot had been hatched to overthrow him.

Four years previously, one General Malet had been committed to prison, being considered of unstable mind. Whilst still under the confinement of the police, Malet formed an audacious plan which was to come within a hair's breadth of success. Being given some writing materials from a kindly guard, by want of forceful ingenuity he was able to execute a forged paper, purporting to be a decree from the Senate, announcing officially the death of the Emperor on Russian fields. This fiction also announced the abolition of the Imperial government, and the establishment of a provisional committee of administration which was to include Malet himself. With this paper, Malet thus secured his own release from prison, and, soon commanding a battalion of troops, made for the Hôtel de Ville, there to prepare reception for the new administration. The plot was eventually foiled and Malet duly tried and shot, but when Napoleon heard this news he rejoiced not. The existence of the plot at all was what concerned him. He had conspired against superiors in former times himself and knew full well that where there was one plot there were generally others. Malet's audacity alone was bound to have pointed out the possibility of success. And the words of the report filled him with dread. "The Emperor had died on Russian fields." How many Parisians had heard the proclamation of those fateful words? And how each day longer he spent on Russian soil brought the echo of those words more credibility. Napoleon saw at once what he must do. He must leave the Grand Armée and return post-haste to Paris.

HEILIGENSTADT

FOR MY BROTHERS KARL AND BEETHOVEN

Oh you men who think or say that I am malevolent, stubborn, or misanthropic, how greatly do you wrong me. You do not know the secret cause which makes me seem that way to you. From childhood on, my heart and soul have been full of the tender feeling of goodwill, and I was ever inclined to accomplish great things. But, think that for six years now I have been hopelessly afflicted, made worse by senseless physicians, from year to year deceived with hopes of improvement, finally compelled to face the prospect of *a lasting malady* (whose cure will take years or, perhaps, be impossible.) Though born with a fiery, active temperament, even susceptible to the diversions of society, I was soon compelled to withdraw myself, to live life alone. If at times I tried to forget all this, oh how harshly was I flung back by the doubly sad experience of my bad hearing. Yet it was impossible for me to say to people, 'Speak louder, shout, for I am deaf.' Ah, how could I possibly admit an infirmity in the *one sense* which ought to be more perfect in me than in others, a sense which I once possessed in the highest perfection, a perfection such as few in my profession enjoy or ever have enjoyed. - Oh I cannot do it; therefore forgive me when you see me draw back when I would have gladly mingled with you. My misfortune is doubly painful to me because I am bound to be misunderstood; for me there can be no relaxation with my fellow men, no refined conversations, no mutual exchange of ideas. I must live alone, like one who has been banished; I can mix with society only as much as true necessity demands. If I approach near to people, a hot terror seizes upon me, and I fear being exposed to the danger that my condition might be noticed. Thus it has been during the last six months which I have spent in the country. By ordering me to spare my hearing as much as possible, my intelligent doctor almost fell in with my own present frame of mind, though sometimes I ran counter to it by yielding to my desire for companionship. But what a humiliation for me when someone standing next to me heard a flute in the distance and *I heard nothing*, or someone heard a *shepherd singing* and again I heard nothing. Such incidents drove me almost to despair; a little more of that and I would have ended my life - it was only *my art* that held me back. Ah, it seemed to me impossible to leave the world until I had brought forth all that I felt was within me. So I endured this wretched existence - truly wretched for so susceptible a body, which can be thrown by a sudden change from the best condition to the very worst. - *Patience*, they say, is what I now choose for my guide, and I have done so - I hope my determination will remain firm to endure until it pleases the inexorable Fates to break the thread. Perhaps I shall get better, perhaps not; I am ready. - Forced to become a philosopher already in my twenty-eighth year, - oh it is not easy, and for the artist much more difficult than for anyone else. - Divine One, thou seest my innermost soul; thou knowest that therein dwells the love of mankind and the desire to do good. - Oh fellow men, when at some point you read this, consider then that you have done me an injustice; someone who has had misfortune may console himself to find a similar case to his, who despite all the limitations of Nature nevertheless did everything within his powers to become accepted among worthy artists and men. - You, my brothers Karl and, as soon as I am dead, if Dr. Schmidt is still alive, ask him in my name to describe my malady, and attach this written document to his account of my illness so that so far as is possible at least the world may become reconciled to me after my death. - At the same time, I declare you two to be the heirs to my small fortune (if so it can be called); divide it fairly; bear with and help each other. What injury you have done me you know was long ago forgiven. To you, brother Karl, I give special thanks for the attachment you have shown me of late. It is my wish that you may have a better and freer life than I have had. Recommend *virtue* to your children; it alone, not money, can make them happy. I speak from experience; this was what upheld me in time of misery. Thanks to it and to my art, I did not end my life by suicide. - Farewell and love each other. - I thank all my friends, particularly *Prince Lichnowsky* and *Professor Schmidt* - I would like the instruments from Prince L. to be preserved by one of you, but not to be the cause of strife between you, and as soon as they can serve you a better purpose, then sell them. How happy I shall be if I can still be helpful to you in my grave - so be it; - With joy I hasten to meet death. - If it comes before I have had the chance to develop all my artistic capacities, it will still be coming too soon despite my harsh fate, and I should probably wish it later - yet even so I should be happy, for would it not free me from a state of endless suffering? - Come when thou wilt, I shall meet thee bravely. - Farewell and do not wholly forget me when I am still dead; I deserve this from you, for during my lifetime I was thinking of you often and of ways to make you happy - please be so -

Heilgnstadt
Ludwig van Beethoven
6 October
1802   (Located here in the original is a big ink stain)

As you can see, Beethoven wrote the above in 1802. When he wrote it, he was thirty two. It's called the Heiligenstadt Testament, predictably enough, because he wrote it in a place called Heiligenstadt. Heiligenstadt was a village about an hour and a half's coach journey outside the walls of Imperial Vienna. Where is it now? Well, what do you know; it's a railway station in modern

Vienna itself *(2009 Multimap.)* So let's return to imagining Heiligenstadt's a village in 1802.

What does the Heiligenstadt Testament mean? It's a letter written by a composer about going deaf. Right? *Right.* What else? He's very upset about it. Right? *Right.* So, it's all pretty straight forward. If you think the Heiligenstadt Testament is straight forward, then go straight forward to the next chapter. Otherwise, read on...

Extracts of HEILIGENSTADT TESTAMENT, including last page

1. Don't forget the ink stain. The ink stain is like the world's biggest full stop. This is a letter with a distinct air of finality about it.

2. Look at the original of the Heiligenstadt Testament. The handwriting is measured and even. Beethoven is calm and considered. He has thought about what he is saying before he has sat down to write it. He's not in the grip of inspiration, his heart isn't pounding. There's no crisis in the writing itself, but the writing relates a crisis. Beethoven knows the score.

3. *What is the score?*
3a. Resignation to a painful future. The letter is almost a suicide note, but it isn't. It's an affirmation of life's purpose despite adversity. Nevertheless, death stalks Beethoven throughout. The man writing this is profoundly aware of his own mortality.

3b. "With joy I hasten to meet death." Why does Beethoven seem to think death so imminent? I think this is an *imagination of death* that made him *live* thereafter to the full. This *imagination of death* transformed him. There is an *imaginative* difference between the 2nd and 3rd symphonies for example, and the Heiligenstadt Testament was written between them. The difference is huge. The loss of a faculty (and especially one as crucial to Beethoven as his hearing) made Beethoven crucially aware parts of himself were starting to fail. It is this awareness that makes Beethoven strive towards musical *immortality* thereafter.

3c. Beethoven says at the start of the letter that he has been aware of going deaf for six years. Then he starts to romanticise his own condition. "I was soon compelled to withdraw myself..." He makes it sound as if he's been going deaf virtually all his life, almost since childhood. He has been compelled "to live life alone." This romanticisation of Beethoven's condition is not simple exaggeration. By imagining that he has been deaf for longer than he has been deaf, Beethoven is also imagining how he will be deafer for longer than he has already been deaf in the future. Beethoven extends his deafness towards childhood because he sees an increasingly silent future stretching out before him. At some point, I think, he *imagines his own death as a composer* because of this (this is another reason he is so preoccupied by physical death, which is acting, partially at least, as a metaphor.) "A little more of that and I would have ended my life - it was only *my art* that held me back."

3d. *There's something else here*. It is not physical death that frightens Beethoven. It is the *living death* of not being able to compose. And then, a triumph! "Ah, it seemed to me impossible to leave the world until I had brought forth all that I felt was within me." His art, here, is not a hindrance, *it is also the reason he survives!* It is pushing him forward. He must, *somehow*, go on. *He must continue!*

4. *Did Beethoven have a problem about his age?* In the Heiligenstadt Testament, he says he's twenty seven. We know he was thirty two. Is there guile in this, or was Beethoven simply confused? Or with sleight of pen was he awarding himself a greater precocity than he merited? Or did Beethoven actually write the Heiligenstadt Testament in 1797 and for some reason date it 1802? *I don't know*. But I think we've already established that anything to do with Beethoven, days and dates can quickly turn into endless confusion. *Let's not pursue this one any further.*

5. Why does Beethoven miss his brother Johann's name out of the initial title to the letter, and later on in the letter too? *I don't know* and I've never read a convincing

explanation. There's nothing to suggest that in October 1802 Beethoven and Johann were having a row, for example. Most scholars simply ignore this one, and treat the letter as if Johann's name was there anyway. *I'm going to do the same.*

6. "Great men", wrote Marguerite Yourcenar of the Roman Emperor Hadrian, "are characterised precisely by the extreme position which they take, and their heroism consists in holding to that extremity throughout their lives." All I can say is the mind that wrote that is warped. If you follow the logic of this statement through, you come to the conclusion that the more extreme you are, the greater you are. This can't be right. *So let's look at it another way.* Extreme positions do not have to be *taken up*. They can be *forced on us*, in which case our greatness, or more correctly I think, our triumph, corresponds to the way in which we respond to living subject to whatever adversity we have no choice but to learn to deal with. With Beethoven, this adversity, this extremity, was deafness. He didn't choose it, it was forced on him. *He had to live with this throughout his life*, or at least, live with the full realisation of it throughout his life subsequent of the Heiligenstadt Testament. His extreme position was to continue. Not to continue living, but to *continue living as a deaf composer*. Never forget that. It is an act of the uttermost courage. And there is more than one way in which Beethoven had no choice. He had no choice about going deaf, but he also had no choice about being a deaf composer. If you're musical, and you're going deaf, you would have thought you'd start to consider some pretty serious career changes. Well, Beethoven did. And he came to the conclusion that the affliction of deafness meant that other musical options he might have had, such as being a travelling piano virtuoso for instance (a concert pianist in today's language) , or a Kappelmeister (nearest modern equivalent a conductor), were denied

to him. And music was the only thing Beethoven knew. The family was musical, and he'd been trained in music since he was knee high to a harpsichord. So when Beethoven searched around for a career change, *being a deaf composer was the best* (or least bad) *option he possessed*. From which we arrive at a paradox. It is not so much that deafness constricted Beethoven's capacity to compose. *It is the very fact of deafness that turned Beethoven into a truly dedicated composer in the first place.*

6a. *Let's follow this through further.* In 1802, Beethoven had yet to write virtually any of the music for which he is now best known. The 3rd Symphony was a year away, and obviously, numbers Four to Nine lay in the future. He had yet to write his opera *Fidelio*. He had yet to write the Violin Concerto. He had yet to write three of the five piano concertos. True, he had written the *Moonlight* piano sonata, but he had yet to write the *Waldstein*, the *Appassionata*, or *Das Lebewohl*, or the *Hammerklavier*. Admittedly, in total, of the thirty two piano sonatas, by 1802 he had in fact already written twenty, but I'm not really contradicting myself here. *He hadn't written most of the ones for which he is now best known.* And besides, it stands to reason that the young Beethoven was likely to write a lot of piano sonatas before he tried writing concertos, symphonies, or operas. Beethoven was a pianist, after all! In general, the point holds good. In 1802, Beethoven had written only six of the sixteen string quartets, and none of the last five, which are generally considered the most significant. He was still a year away from writing the *Kreutzer* sonata, and he hadn't written the *Archduke* piano trio, and he hadn't written the *Missa Solemnis* either.

6b. If you're getting worried about references to lots of pieces of music you haven't heard, don't. It's the intention of this novel to confine all you really need to know about Beethoven to the *Moonlight* Piano Sonata, the 3rd Symphony, and the 9th Symphony, all references to which should appear self-explanatory as need arises.

6c. If at any point you don't find 6b. to be true, then write to me via my publisher (but don't expect your money back).

6d. You don't need even to have heard the three pieces of music listed in 6b. to follow all this. But, come on! Show some curiosity. Go out and buy copies! Or, if you're hard up, go and tape them from your local library.

7. If you listen to any decent piece of Beethoven written after 1802 with both your ears working well, I hope you'll notice the following. There will at some point be a prolonged rising crescendo which seems to say *things are going to get better, they really are*. This crescendo will then be followed by a development of a sequence of falling chords in direct contradiction to the spirit of *things are going to get better, they really are*. The sequence of falling chords will categorically state *things can only get worse*. The first movement of the 3rd Symphony is a classic in this regard. Another paradox and one again related to living the life of a deaf composer. Beethoven passionately believed that the condition of humankind could improve. And yet his own condition, his own deafness, only ever got worse.

8. *Who was Professor Schmidt?* Dr. Johann Schmidt was Beethoven's doctor, and Professor of Medicine at Vienna University. Dr. Schmidt, the "intelligent doctor", was the reason Beethoven was in Heiligenstadt in the first place, and the only physician Beethoven ever fully trusted. The choice of Dr. Schmidt is indicative of how little Beethoven trusted established experts on deafness because ears were not what Dr. Schmidt was about. Dr.

Schmidt was an eye specialist. Dr. Schmidt advised Beethoven to try and save his hearing by going on *quiet* restoratives to the countryside as a means of escaping the *noise* of Vienna. *Noise*, Dr. Schmidt theorised, was likely to make Beethoven's deafness worse.

8a. Whether Dr. Schmidt's theory was true or not, by advising Beethoven to spend as much time in Heiligenstadt as possible, he was doing Beethoven a favour. The countryside around Heiligenstadt is the countryside which inspired the Sixth, *Pastoral*, Symphony.

8b. *Loud, banging noises* were the worst. Another paradox. As Beethoven's deafness increased, so *loud, banging noises* became the only ones he could reliably hear. Beethoven died when he was fifty seven. But even relatively early, when he was thirty six, this was already a problem. *How do we know?* Because the Violin Concerto, written in 1806, starts with four drum beats. No one had ever started a concerto or symphony with drum beats before. As Beethoven sat in the concert hall, the four drum beats helped him know when the Violin Concerto was beginning. We can extend this principle throughout a listening of Beethoven. The same paradox in a slightly different form comes back at us time and time again. *When Beethoven is most conscious of his deafness, his music is at its loudest.* He seems to first become conscious of this paradox himself in 1802. The incidental but delightful seven variations on the theme of *God Save The King* (WoO.78) date from this year. The last piano chord of these is quite *deafeningly* loud.

8c. *Did Beethoven have any other doctors?* Yes, several, all of whom he considered to be quacks. Some of them probably were. But before 1802, Beethoven seems to have considered any doctor who couldn't cure his deafness a quack anyway. And so we can deduce that prior to 1802, Beethoven must have been living in a state of *profound nervous anxiety*, running from one doctor to another, seeking words of clean-bill-of-hearing-health with which he could temporarily delude himself.

8d. *So what was different about Dr. Schmidt?* Dr. Schmidt had empathy with Beethoven's predicament. And what was different was 1802. In 1802, Beethoven resigned himself to the fact that his deafness would only ever increase. That is, fundamentally, one of the things the Heiligenstadt Testament definitely tells us. I think this resignation to deafness was a distinct spiritual improvement on the state of *profound nervous anxiety* that had preceded it.

8e. The *profound nervous anxiety* had been profound indeed. Beethoven, despairing of "senseless physicians", had even taken to a "faith healing" priest, one Pater Weiss of the Metropolitan Church of St. Stephen. As well as the laying on of hands, Weiss claimed to be familiar with the physiology of the ear, but whether he was or he wasn't, Weiss couldn't do Beethoven's ears any good.

8f. *In the light of modern medical science, what theories have been put forward to explain Beethoven's deafness?* The answer is a very great many, and, unless you're an ear specialist, they don't enlighten you very much. Nevertheless, it seems probable that at least originally; Beethoven suffered from some kind of tinnitus in his left ear. When the ringing of the tinnitus departed, it seems his hearing was much impaired. When exactly the deafness extended to his right ear isn't known. There have been various diagnoses linking his deafness with a 1796 illness caused by Beethoven coming home on a very hot day, immediately undressing, and cooling himself in the draft of an open window. And there's the story that Beethoven, refusing to play for French officers who occupied Vienna in 1805, walked alone from Grätz to Troppau in the rain, aggravating his deafness by a heavy cold. And then there's the story that Beethoven much aggravated his deafness by throwing himself to the ground in a rage and fury around 1810. And there have also been theories revolving around a typhoid infection. The last is probably the most plausible. In 1964, Dr. A. Laskiewicz diagnosed "*neuritis acoustica* after typhoid fever... smallpox, repeated head colds and influenza."

8g. *Does 8f. matter?* All advances in human comprehension matter. But obviously, modern medical science didn't help Beethoven much.

8h. *What did help Beethoven?* The countryside around Heiligenstadt. And ear horns. *A bit*. These were predominantly made by one Joseph Nepomuk Maelzel. Maelzel was a Viennese mechanic and inventor, operating in Vienna under the title of Court Mechanician. Maelzel was part Thomas Edison, part Phineas T. Barnum, and part fraudster. He invented ingenious mechanical appliances of all kinds, by which he profited hugely in an age that adored clocks run by steam and contraptions that could rise as if by magic into the air (the balloon was as new as a space rocket in 1960). Beethoven was fascinated by Maelzel's workshops. Maelzel invented the Metronome, which he persuaded Beethoven publicly recommend. As in, *"The new Metronome! A miraculous musical time keeper! As recommended by the fêted composer Ludwig van Beethoven!"* Maelzel made a fortune out of the metronome. Beethoven didn't. Nevertheless, the second *Allegretto* movement of the Eighth Symphony was inspired by the metronome's regularity. *Tick, tick, tick*, or "ta ta ta lieber lieber Maelzel" as Beethoven composed a song. Maelzel also invented the Panharmonicon, a most ingenious device that could mechanically imitate several instruments of the orchestra, such as the trombone, the clarinet, the viola and the cello. The Panharmonicon caused a sensation in Vienna, as did Maelzel's Mechanical Trumpeter, which blew an Austrian military march via clockwork driven bellows. There was nothing Maelzel felt he couldn't invent, and what he couldn't invent, he stole or faked. He claimed, for example, to have invented a Mechanical Chess Player, which was actually constructed by one Kempelen, of whom sadly, little else is known. In any case, the Mechanical Chess Player was a fake. When the Emperor Napoleon was camped at Schönbrunn, outside Vienna, in 1809, he played a game against this machine and was much impressed. Luckily for Maelzel, the Emperor did not discover there was a man concealed inside.

8i. *Why didn't ear horns help Beethoven more?* Because he didn't like using them. Why? *How would you feel with the end of a trumpet sticking out of your ear?*

8j. Dr. Schmidt died in 1809, which upset Beethoven greatly. He was replaced by Dr. Johann Malfatti, who, like Dr. Schmidt, recommended the quiet of the countryside. But Dr. Malfatti clearly thought further afield than his predecessor. It is on Dr. Malfatti's recommendation that Beethoven first went to Teplitz, in the August of 1811.

9. *Who were Karl and Johann?* They were Beethoven's brothers, of course! *Yes, but who were they?* Their full names were Kaspar Karl and Nikolaus Johann. Karl was four years younger than Beethoven, and would die twelve years before him in 1815. Nikolaus was six years younger than Beethoven, and outlived him by nine years. Karl was a bank official. Nikolaus worked as a chemist's assistant in Vienna until 1808, when he

bought his own pharmacy in Linz, and became wealthy, largely as a result of war profiteering during Napoleon's occupation of Vienna in 1809 which resulted in shortages of all kinds, including drugs. Eventually, Johann bought an estate in Gneixendorf, and took to signing himself "Landowner." Beethoven wrote back signing himself "Brainowner."

10. *Who was Prince Lichnowsky?* Prince Karl Lichnowsky was a friend and the first patron of Beethoven's, and one time pupil of Mozart. Lichnowsky was one of those jewel like individuals who all people with talent coming from relatively inferior social circumstances need, financially or otherwise, if they are to be allowed to succeed. Lichnowsky used all his influence to promote Beethoven, frequently gave Beethoven use of his private orchestra, and commissioned him to compose many pieces of music. Further, in 1800, perceiving Beethoven's need to compose and yet be financially independent, Lichnowsky granted Beethoven an income of 600 florins a year, an arrangement that lasted until at least 1806.

11. *More on Beethoven's income.* In 1809, Jérôme Bonaparte, Napoleon's youngest brother, and then King of Westphalia, offered Beethoven a very lucrative deal indeed to move from Vienna to the Court of Kassel. Now the Viennese, having just suffered the 1805 French occupation and diplomatic humiliation at the hands of Napoleon (and being just about to suffer the same thing again in 1809) were mighty displeased at the idea of losing their most fêted composer to the Bonaparte family as well. On the other hand, Beethoven was well aware that Mozart had been buried in a paupers' grave, and he was damn sure the same thing wasn't going to happen to him. With real intention or not, Beethoven made all the signs of accepting Jérôme Bonaparte's offer. If the Viennese wanted him to stay, they could

match the deal, one much more lucrative to him than the income he had earlier been granted by Lichnowsky. Three other noblemen agreed to provide Beethoven with a regular income for the rest of his life. The three were Prince Ferdinand Kinsky, the Archduke Rudolph (the Emperor Franz's brother and ecclesiastic, to whom the *Hammerklavier* Piano Sonata is dedicated), and Prince Franz Maximilian Lobkowitz, who together promised Beethoven 4000 florins per annum. With this Beethoven was hardly rich, but he was comfortable. On the 1st of March 1809, the Princes' Decree announced:

As it is proven... that man cannot entirely devote himself to his art except in the condition of being free from all material care, and that it is only in this way that he can produce those great and elevated works that are the glory of art, the undersigned are resolved to shelter Herr Ludwig van Beethoven from need.

There were some problems with this allowance, most notably caused by Napoleon's second occupation of Vienna in 1809. Napoleon demanded a levy of fifty million francs from the Austrians to withdraw, which, along with later battles against Napoleon, helped to almost bankrupt the Austrian aristocracy and devalue the currency by four fifths by 1815. However, the Prince's ultimately kept their word, and the allowance was index linked. This act of farsighted generosity is to my knowledge one of the first examples of long term public subsidy of any artist, and what a good idea it was. For 4000 florins at 1809 prices a year, the Prince's secured about half of Beethoven's entire works, almost two centuries of orchestras found employment, and a great many record companies have made an absolute fortune (and, since both records and CDs are made of plastic, a great many oil companies must have profited handsomely over the years as well). In taxation alone, this 4000 florins a year must have been repaid to the

Austrian exchequer and the exchequers of the rest of the world many thousands of times over. *Moral; Subsidy, wisely given, is more properly public investment, and far more analogous to Research and Development than with charity handouts.* "But, ah" goes the sceptic, "not every artist is Beethoven." And I would argue in reply that very few are ever given the chance to prove they could be.

12. *What else happened in 1802?* After the then General Napoleon Bonaparte's earlier victories against the Austrians at Marengo and Hohenlinden, France's power in Continental Europe was further consolidated by the Concordat with Rome by which Pope Pius VII recognised the French Republic. In other words, the Vatican admitted that the French Revolution had happened, and wasn't going to go away. Given that Napoleon wanted the Pope to attend his Coronation in 1804, this is just as well.

In 1802 France signed the peace treaty of Amiens with a war-weary England. By this treaty, England gained recognition in Ceylon and Trinidad, but relinquished Egypt, Malta and the Cape of Good Hope. France agreed to evacuate Naples (which probably has some bearing on Giulietta Guicciardi's decision to move there the following year). In 1802, Napoleon Bonaparte was elected First Consul of the French Republic for life. In 1802, Napoleon Bonaparte first suffered from stomach cramps.

In 1802 in England, the Prime Minister Henry Addington was deeply unpopular for signing the treaty of Amiens, and William Wordsworth published *Milton! Thou shouldst be living at this hour* (Milton had in fact been dead for one 128 years.) Wordsworth considered England "a fen/Of stagnant waters", full of "selfish men."

Michael Black

In 1802 in Bath, England, Jane Austen was writing *Sense and Sensibility*. She had begun writing it in 1797, and it was to take her another nine years. You would have thought this was some kind of a record, but it isn't (read on.) *Sense and Sensibility* has nothing to do with the French revolution, nothing to do treaty of Amiens, and nothing to do with Napoleonic wars which tore Europe apart throughout most of Jane Austen's life time. These observations hold generally true of all Jane Austen's novels. *They have nothing to do with the Napoleonic wars whatsoever.* Except that, in all of them it will be discovered there is a remarkable shortage of eligible young men.

In Weimar in 1802, the novelist (and dramatist, and poet, anatomist, botanist, politician and geologist) Johann Wolfgang von Goethe was still working on his version of *Faust*. He had started working on it in 1775, and didn't finish it until 1832. This must be something of a record, albeit an egg-bound one, and to my knowledge it is.

In 1832, at Abbotsford in Scotland, Sir Walter Scott died. Sir Walter Scott was by far the most famous novelist of his age. Scott was also the writer of the first widely and internationally read *Life of Napoleon*, and saved the Scottish pound note and the Scottish deerhound from extinction in his spare time. In his unspare time, Sir Walter Scott single handedly invented the historical novel, and thus inspired Alexander Pushkin, Victor Hugo, Honoré de Balzac, Alexander Dumas, James Fenimore Cooper and many more since. Without Scott, Tolstoy's *War and Peace* is impossible. In *War and Peace*, it will be discovered there are some rather fine descriptions of the Russian's campaign of attrition against Napoleon in 1812. Tolstoy's hero is General Kutusov, who he sees as perfecting the scorched earth policy. *But that's another story.*

So's this. In 1832, in England, the Great Reform Act passed through the Houses of Parliament. The Great Reform Act enfranchised the mercantile middle classes of England, who, due to the industrial revolution, were a growing body of opinion most urgently requiring representation. Many historians have seen the Great Reform Act as one of the principle reasons that, unlike virtually the rest of Europe, Britain had no revolution between 1789 and 1917. Sir Walter Scott apparently loathed the idea of the Great Reform Act, and loathed the idea of the French revolution as well, at least in retrospect. Presumably with Napoleon in mind, "the hour has come" he concluded, "but not the man." Scott, quoting Horace whilst returning through Macclesfield from his last trip to the Continent in 1832, is said to have uttered "Odi profanum vulgus et arceo" which means "I loathe the vulgar crowd, and I shun them" but I don't believe Sir Walter would ever say such a thing. Anyone who can write characters such as Jeanie Deans in *The Heart of Midlothian* is a man of the people, and history books can lie. In fact some of them I wouldn't touch with a barge-pole, which I believe to be a Macclesfield expression.

In Austria in 1802, one Antonie Brentano was described as being "like a glass of water that has been left to stand for too long" (read on). Also, the Emperor Francis appointed Prince Clemens Lothar Wenzel von Metternich to the post of Austrian Ambassador to Saxony at Dresden. Prince Metternich would subsequently become Austrian Ambassador to France, where, deftly, he saw fit to gain French intelligence by sleeping with Napoleon's favourite sister Pauline, one of the great classical beauties of her age and a famed nymphomaniac to boot. Napoleon had two other sisters, Elize and Caroline. Whether Prince von Metternich also slept with them is not known, but where Prince von

Metternich is concerned, most things are possible. Most things, that is, except revolutions. Like Sir Walter Scott, Metternich loathed them. In fact, it is true to say Metternich spent a diplomatic lifetime suppressing them. Whilst Ambassador to France, Prince von Metternich was also the architect of the marriage between the by now Emperor Napoleon and the Austrian royal princess, Marie-Louise, but here we are stretching our narrative apace to 1810. Ultimately, Prince von Metternich was the chief architect of the Congress of Vienna of 1815, which concluded the post-Napoleonic European settlement, by which the old order of Europe re-established itself, and by which a great many of the dreams of the French Revolution were destroyed forever. Or rather, *so far...*

And in 1815, Prince von Metternich did more than run the Congress of Vienna. He also ran the Viennese secret police. On the 12th July 1815, at the height of the Congress of Vienna, one of the police reports is on Josephine Deym, *née* von Brunsvik. It reads "the morality of the Countess does not appear to enjoy a good reputation, and it is stated that she cannot be absolved from having given grounds for conjugal quarrels." Josephine had, at the very least, by this time had an affair with one Count Wolkenstein. Von Stackelburg, her second husband, had by this time upped it to pursue an illusory fortune in Russia. He took the three children Josephine bore him, Laura, Theophile and Minona. Josephine pleaded "Let me have the children. I have borne them in pain." But Von Stackelburg took them anyway.

In the summer of 1815, due to the Congress, Vienna was awash with foreign diplomats and dignitaries of all kinds. It was awash with parties and balls, and it was awash with sexual *frisson*. Josephine and her sister Therese had suspected they were subject to police attentions as early as 1802. This is possibly connected to the sister's association with Beethoven. Beethoven had some very powerful friends, but was subject to police attentions himself, and was once arrested on a charge of public vagrancy. In the police cell, no one would believe who he said he was:

POLICEMAN   What's your name then?
BEETHOVEN   What?
POLICEMAN   *(shouting)* What's your name?
BEETHOVEN   Oh. Beethoven
POLICEMAN   Oh is it now? And my name's Mozart
BEETHOVEN   What?
POLICEMAN   *(shouting)* My name's Mozart
BEETHOVEN   No it's not
   You can imagine the rest.

13. *The Heiligenstadt Testament is very melancholy. Is Beethoven's melancholy a symptom only of his deafness?* No. It represents more than that. It represents a romantic condition as well, the syndrome of the *artist-outside-conventional-society*, but in Beethoven's case, this outside-ness was forced on him, or so he would have us believe. Thus Beethoven laments the extent of his isolation.

13a. *Do we really believe this?* Hard to say. The life of a composer, deaf or not, is isolated by its very nature. What is certain is that Beethoven's deafness made him more isolated than he had been previously. This is probably another way of saying he was more isolated than he wanted to be.

13b. *Was Beethoven really isolated?* In one sense, no. He had lots of very understanding friends and patrons. A great deal of Beethoven's isolation was largely in his own head (or ears). This should not be read, however, as making isolation any less isolating.

13c. *More on melancholy*. What is romantic melancholy, and *why is it different from what we would now call clinical depression?* I think the difference is melancholia loves itself, whereas depression doesn't. That is to say melancholia is potentially creative, whereas depression is simply depressing. WARNING: JUST BECAUSE MELANCHOLIA CAN BE CREATIVE, DO NOT TRY IT!!! MELANCHOLIA, LIKE DEPRESSION, CAN ALSO LEAD TO SUICIDE.

13d. *You want proof?* Take Johann Wolfgang von Goethe's hero Werther. Werther and Beethoven have a great deal in common. When Goethe published *The Sorrows of Young Werther* in 1774, he was twenty four. It immediately catapulted him into European literary stardom. It also caused a scandal, being seen by many as a justification of adultery and suicide (activities in the popular mind not previously closely connected.) Goethe feigned modesty, but loved every minute of it. Widely regarded as the first tragic novel in European literature, *The Sorrows of Young Werther* tells the tale of how Werther falls in love with Charlotte, who is betrothed to Albert. Werther gives himself up to Charlotte whilst Albert is away. When Albert comes back, Werther tears himself away, and takes a provincial job as a lawyer (if you're in any doubt here, read *spiritual death.*) He tries to forget Charlotte, but fails miserably. Werther takes to a country retreat, like Beethoven after him. Eventually, knowing no hope of salvation from longing or pain, Werther kills himself. Werther was a hero for his time. Werther helped make the *Romeo and Juliet* the most performed Shakespeare of his day, Romeo's fate mirroring Werther's own.

The Sorrows of Young Werther is the first European novel of loneliness, the first novel to emotionally aggrandise isolation. And it set a romantic trend of heroicising both. The book was translated into every major European language. Ladies wore Werther jewellery. There was Werther porcelain, Werther paintings and Werther plays and operas by the score. There were even several Werther imitation suicides. Werther became an archetypal romantic hero, seeing suicide as more noble than any kind of accidental death, or even, in many ways, death in battle (this is the tradition that insists Shelley did not die of drowning in an Italian boating accident, but abandoned himself heroically to the seas.)

By the time Beethoven came to write the Heiligenstadt Testament, this tradition of epic suicide was *de rigeur*. And whilst Beethoven ultimately resists Werther's fate, we can note that he makes no bones about contemplating it. Far from the rest of the world seeing Beethoven as weak for so doing, to Beethoven, the contemplation of suicide confirmed his elementally valuable status in his own eyes. As he had the right to *create* himself, so he has the right to *destroy* himself if he so chooses, and either way, he remains in charge of himself (I think there are serious flaws in this argument, but never mind.) Further, Beethoven reconfirms his elemental valuableness by emphasising his loneliness and isolation. *The Sorrows of Young Werther* is epistolary, but comprises only Werther's own letters, and no replies. *Werther was essentially writing letters to himself*. There's at least a possibility with the Letter to the Immortal Beloved and with the Heiligenstadt Testament that Beethoven was doing much the *same thing*. And one other similarity can be noted between Werther and Beethoven too. *The Sorrows of Young Werther* established a romantic tradition that saw unhappy or unrequited or unfulfilled love as in some way more heightened or valid than fulfilled and happy love. *Isolation maketh the man*. Werther is the third person on the outside looking in on the fulfilled love of Albert and Charlotte. Note how this pattern constantly repeated itself in Beethoven's life also. With all the women Beethoven had any kind of romance with, Beethoven is always the outsider, the third person looking in at someone else's marriage or *d'alliance*. Beethoven is always the aspirer to female love, but never the instigator of a secure union.

14. There is an addendum to the Heiligenstadt Testament, dated four days after the main body you have already read. It reads:

Heilgnstadt, 10 October 1802

Thus I bid thee farewell - and indeed sadly. - Yes, that fond hope - which I brought here with me, to be cured to a degree at last - this I must now wholly abandon. As the leaves of autumn fall and are withered - so likewise has my hope been blighted - I leave here - almost as I came - even the high courage - which often inspired me in the beautiful days of summer - has disappeared - Oh Providence - grant me at last but one day of *pure joy* - it is so long since real joy echoed in my heart - Oh when - Oh when, Oh Divine One - shall I feel it again in the temple of nature and of mankind - Never? - No - Oh that would be too hard.

14a. The Addendum reveals that the Beethoven of the main letter was not so resigned to the circumstance of increasing deafness as might have been previously presumed. *The Sorrows of Young Beethoven.* Here he really has relinquished "that fond hope ... to be cured to a degree." In the Addendum he has resigned himself to the fact that the clarity of his former hearing has gone forever. *Why? How?* In other words, *what happened to*

Beethoven in the intervening four days between the main letter and the Addendum?

14b. *Here's one interpretation.* It is autumn, the summer has gone. With it, Beethoven's hopes of restoration fall away. We can imagine him walking around Heiligenstadt during these four days, watching leaves fall all around him. Colours fade as Nature shrivels and seemingly dies. The days grow shorter. Death - and increasingly *silence* - stalks him. And then in desperation some cry of hope, or at least, of desire. "Oh Providence - grant me at last but one day of *pure joy*."

14c. *This is a very great deal to continue to live for*, and Beethoven's ideas of joy were exalted indeed. This desire to find *pure joy* proved sufficient to live on for another twenty five years, and became the means towards self-regeneration. It is not in Providence Beethoven found *pure joy*, but in the act of his own composing. The last movement of the 9th Symphony is a choral rendition of Friedrich von Schiller's *Ode to Joy*. Anthony Burgess's idea of Heaven was the last movement of Beethoven's 9th Symphony playing forever. *Precisely*, and it was Beethoven's Heaven-sent task to compose it in the first place.

14d. "Grant me at last but one day of *pure joy*." I repeat it because it stands repetition. *Forever!* This is the cry of a man effectively inventing hope out of nowhere. *Where did the hope come from? And what is hope?* Hope, I think, is a *remembered future*.

The hope of a *remembered future* of return and restoration is all the Children of Israel had to sustain them in exile for example. Beethoven's hope is not only "one day of *pure joy*." It is also the *remembered future* of his lost hearing. *He finds a way of continuing as a deaf composer by utilising the memory of his almost perfect hearing when younger.* Essentially, out of deafness Beethoven conjures a miracle, a miracle more miraculous than any conquest of war, however grand, can ever be.

Crossing Out The Emperor

INCOGNITO

Napoleon made his own plans for departure. Three sledges were provided, the first prepared to carry Napoleon and Caulaincourt, whose title as the Duke of Vicenza the Emperor proposed to assume whilst travelling incognito, although their figures were strikingly dissimilar, Caulaincourt being tall and raw-boned. But no one present saw fit to question the Emperor's plans. You didn't tell the Emperor Napoleon he was shorter and fatter than the travelling companion he was intent on pretending to be. And neither did Caulaincourt register any reservations about being reduced to the role of valet to himself. The Chief of Staff Berthier was to be left behind, separated from Napoleon for the first time in sixteen years. Upon realising this he protested vehemently, but Napoleon explained he was relying on Berthier's continued presence to maintain continuity with the troops. Although he fully realised what an honour it would be to travel in the Emperor's exclusive company for so long a journey, he was sure Berthier could see where his duties lay. Berthier looked at Caulaincourt, Caulaincourt looked at the ceiling. Berthier instructed his amanuensis to record his Emperor's observation for posterity.

There was a general audience, at which were present General Murat, Eugène and Marshal Ney. The Emperor appointed Murat as head of the Grande Armée in his absence, and promised to return with a fresh army of 1,200,000 men he would raise once he again reached Paris. He assured all present to have no fear, for the Russian pursuit was but temporary. Nor need they fear Prussian retribution as they marched westwards, for his new army would keep his reluctant Germanic allies well in line. No one dared ask Napoleon exactly where his new army was to come from.

Of the Austrians also he assured the assembled company there was no threat. After all, was he, the Emperor Napoleon, not married to the Emperor of Austria's daughter? There followed a happy nodding of diplomatic heads, for here was an incontrovertible fact about which all could agree. As to the ramifications of the marriage, if such had been discussed, there would still have been much rancour, but *that the Emperor was married*, and *to whom*, there could be no disagreement whatsoever. Napoleon then ordered Marshal Ney to Vilnius to reorganize the army, and to strike in all due course such a blow as would discourage further Cossack advance. Lastly, the Emperor wished his audience safe winter quarters westwards beyond the River Niemen. He then took their affectionate farewell, adding how pleased he was to leave them in such fine and courageous spirits. Finally, the Emperor Napoleon departed from Smorgoni at the late hour of ten o'clock at night. It was the 5th of December 1812, and he planned to be back in Paris before Christmas.

The sledges travelled as fast as the weather allowed. The first for Napoleon and Caulaincourt, the second for two officers of rank, the third for one Mameluke Roustan and another anonymous domestic. The sledgers shivered across Lithuania, their plight made all the colder by travelling at first only at night for greater safety, and because all spare clothing was given up to keep the pretend Duke of Vicenza as warm as possible. Caulaincourt suffered particularly in this regard, his master insisting he play the part of valet to perfection. Napoleon found playing the part of someone else had stranger effects than he'd anticipated. He found himself vomiting virtually whatever he ate, and started to wonder as to the real Duke of Vicenza's health. Had he taken on more of his companion's personality than he'd bargained for? He had mad cravings for chocolates and ice cream. Rather like a pregnant woman he thought, before dismissing the notion as utterly ludicrous and beneath him.

Briefly, the thought of rendezvous with the Empress Marie-Louise brought a gallop to his heart, but then the stomach pains which had plagued him throughout the campaign started over again. He still missed Josephine, but what was done was done. There's had been a childless union after all, and Emperors need offspring, and male ones at that. Whatever her sadness, he was sure Josephine understood. He delighted at the thought of seeing his young son again, the infant King of Rome, for whom he had such great plans.

For some time as the sledges battled over the rucks and tranches of the frozen snow, Napoleon found himself comparing Marie-Louise and Josephine in bed. Josephine was the more experienced, and knew the more to please him, and yet there was a familiarity about her that had latterly dampened passion. Marie-Louise on the other hand was all innocence, her delicate fair skin as if untouched. The innocence had always excited him, as did the thought of entry, for it was more than sexual. When Napoleon entered Marie-Louise he was entering into the old aristocracies of Europe, he was uniting the Bonaparte dynasty with that of the ancient Habsburgs! When he entered Marie-Louise, he became the new Charlemagne! When he entered Marie-Louise he became more powerful than the Holy Roman Empire itself! He fell asleep at this pleasing juncture, dozed briefly, and woke up again still thinking of Marie-Louise's fair and delicate skin. And then he dreamed of Josephine again, her unembarrassed boudoir ease such a contrast to the innocent shyness of the new Empress. With Josephine there were no limits, she knew it all. With Marie-Louise it was still rather like walking on egg shells. She still thought of etiquette in bed! How little did she know of rough passion! He smiled to himself as he reflected that what was *ideally* wanted was both of them in bed together. *Jouissance!* Josephine could teach Marie-Louise of all his needs. And then something odd happened. Or rather didn't happen. For the first time in his life, Napoleon found his loins were no longer stirring at the thought of womankind. Not even at the thought of his two favourite women together!

It was odd, and made him question the real Duke of Vicenza's personality still further. And if he was playing Caulaincourt, did the real Caulaincourt know what Napoleon was thinking? Another odd thought. He decided to think no more about it, save to put it down to the cold. But as he felt his loins through his gloves to confirm the absence of any rising, further odd thoughts beset him, each one seemingly odder than the last. He felt he'd put on weight, which seemed an impossibility given the meagreness of his fugitive diet. And so as the sledges sped on, he dismissed the possibility as a delusion. But was this the only delusion, or were there others? For the first time in his life since he was an *étoile* of the military school at Brienne, Napoleon found himself questioning his own judgement. *Very odd indeed*. The Emperor felt strangely ill at ease.

There were several scares, not least at the hamlet of Youpranoni, where the party only narrowly escaped being taken by the Russian partisan Seslavin. And the wolves tracked our travellers relentlessly each night, keeping their distance from the rifles, but only too eager to pounce at the first sign of calamity. Finally, the Emperor incognito and entourage reached Warsaw on the 10th of December 1812. Here they encountered the Abbé de Pradt, then ambassador of France to the Diet of Poland, endeavouring to reconcile the various rumours which poured from every quarter as to his Emperor's and the Grande Armée's welfare. It wasn't outright victory, but that didn't mean it was outright defeat. He had heard from Vilnius of a victory crossing the Beresina, with some 6,000 Russian prisoners taken. This report however lived uneasily with the news of a general withdrawal across the River Niemen, but then the withdrawal could be tactical. The Emperor's strategic genius had often before seemed like foolhardiness until the final acts of the campaign. He was sure the Grande Armée would rise again. The Abbé had just so reassured himself, and practised a summarising speech of the above which he would diplomatically disseminate on the morrow, when a figure like a spectre, wrapped in furs stiffened with hoar-frost, stalked into his apartements, supported, for the figure was most weary, by the anonymous domestic of the third sledge. It was with shock and difficulty that the Abbé recognised the shivering traveller as Caulaincourt, the Duke of Vicenza (the real one.)

"You here, Caulaincourt?!" said the astonished ambassador prelate. "And where is the Emperor?"

"At the Hôtel d'Angleterre, waiting for you."

"Why not stop at the palace?"

"He travels incognito."

"Do you need anything?"

"Some Burgundy or Malaga brandy."

"All is at your service - but whither are you travelling?"

"To Paris."

"To Paris! But where is the army?"

"It no longer exists" said Caulaincourt, looking downwards to the floor.

"And the victory at Beresina - and the 6,000 prisoners?"

"We got across, that is all - the prisoners were a few hundred men, and they escaped. We have had other business than to guard them."

The Abbé de Pradt's curiosity far from satisfied, he hastened to the Hôtel d'Angleterre. In the courtyard stood three sledges in dilapidated condition. The Emperor Napoleon had not travelled on such vehicles, surely?! And where were the horses? The Abbé was just remarking to himself on the seeming absence of stabling facilities, when he was ushered most mysteriously into a back room, where a servant was blowing a fire made of green and incombustible wood. Then he saw the Emperor. He seemed at once both drawn, pale cheeked and yet much plumper than in recent portraits by David or by some rogue-ish copyist. And he seemed to be eating some kind of sweets from an inside pocket. Aniseed, if the aroma was to be believed. "Your Majesty", said the Abbé, wisely limiting himself to formal greetings in such unusual and testing circumstances. "Are you yourself?" It seemed a reasonable question. He had heard of the travel incognito, and here was his Emperor, dressed in a green pelise, covered with lace and lined with furs, and all the while walking agitatedly around the apartment as if to generate from his own movements the warmth the fire refused to create. "Monsieur l'Ambassador!" said Napoleon, turning suddenly round and standing stock still. The greeting seemed one of gaiety, which, given the news he had heard from Caulaincourt, the Abbé found most surprising. And so the Ambassador prelate limited himself once more to formal greetings and ingratiation's as he helped Napoleon off with his cloak.

"Is everything to your Majesty's satisfaction?" he then inquired. Napoleon came closer to the inconstant fire, rubbing his hands vigorously against the flames. To the Abbé they seemed strangely hairless. And he noted silently Napoleon had not asked of his welfare. A sure sign the Emperor had weighty matters on his mind. "I would guess", said the Emperor, at length turning round from the fire, "that the minds of the inhabitants of the

Grand Duchy of Warsaw have been much changed since they were led to believe the Grande Armée would free them from the Russian yoke. And, since they think they cannot be free Polanders, I would assume they are making renewed overtures to Prussia." "Most perspicacious your Majesty" replied the Ambassador.

The entrance of two Polish ministers checked the burgeoning conversation before its deliberations had proceeded further. Caulaincourt had obviously been busy relaying news of the Emperor's arrival. The Emperor's attention turned to the new arrivals immediately. "We must levy ten thousand Poles" he said, "and check the advance of these Russians. The French and the Poles are natural allies against the Muscovite barbarians of the east. A sword and a horse are all that is necessary. There is but a single step between the sublime and the ridiculous." The immediate relevance of this last remark struck the Abbé de Pradt as tangential to say the least, but he let it pass, assuming the mind of Napoleon to be much quicker and more fertile than his own. Clearly, he surmised, there had been set backs, but the mood of the Emperor reassured him nonetheless. At a time of crisis, once more it was clear that Napoleon Bonaparte knew *exactly what to do.*

The two Polish ministers congratulated the Emperor Napoleon on evading so many dangers.

"Dangers!" replied the Emperor, "none in the world. I live for agitation. The more I bustle the better I am. It is for the kings of old Europe to fatten in their palaces - horseback and the fields are for me. Why do I find you so much alarmed, gentlemen?"

"We are at a loss to gather the truth of the news about the Grande Armée" replied the two ministers. The Abbé could only admire the foolhardiness of such a bold observation, for it was the question much on his own mind. But then the ministers had never met Napoleon before.

"Bah!" replied the Emperor. "The Grande Armée is in a superb condition! I have 120,000 men - I have beaten the Russians in every action. The army will recruit anew at Vilnius - I am going to bring up three hundred thousand men - Success will render the Russians foolhardy - I will give them battle once or twice upon the River Oder, and in a month I will be again on the Niemen!"

This was the news of regrouping the Abbé had been waiting for! Whatever the setbacks, to Napoleon's quick and agile mind the future seemed assured. Whereas to any common observer it would seem that by again reaching the Niemen the Emperor would only be marching to the same position he had gained without force the previous spring, in fact it was all part of a master plan to draw Alexander's army and the Cossacks from their snowy lairs! Oh, what genius did France still possess at her helm! The Ambassador moved closer to the fire, as if warmingly reassured.

"I have more weight upon my throne, than at the head of the Grande Armée" said Napoleon, thinking darkly to himself of Malet's conspiracy. He noted the silence of the room that wrapped itself around his words, and mentally observed his own great insight. "Certainly, I quit my soldiers with regret. But I must watch Prussia" he continued. He thought of the Emperor Francis, the father of his beloved Marie-Louise. "And Austria too" he found himself adding. The head of the Habsburgs was an inconstant calculator! Why hadn't he seen it earlier? The Emperor had visions of his alliances unravelling around him in the Russian aftermath. And then his composure settled him once again. The situation was tenuous certainly, but only bold actions could remedy it. Turning abruptly, he fixed the Ambassador's eye.

"I have seen worse affairs than this. All that has happened goes for nothing - a mere misfortune, in which the enemy can claim no credit. It was the weather." Looks of alarm spread across the faces of the two Polish ministers. No less than the independence of Poland depended on Napoleon's success! The Emperor changed his tack. "I beat them everywhere - they wished to cut me off at the Beresina - but I made an ass of them all. I had good troops and cannon - the position was superb - five hundred metres of marsh we trudged across - a river. The river, usually of course it would be of no consequence, but the weather..." The Emperor's voice trailed off, lost in thought. Once more Napoleon felt the cold, and the sickness stirring in his stomach.

"Your Majesty". The Abbé received no answer. "Would your Majesty care for some brandy?" The Abbé poured some anyway. Napoleon sipped at it somewhat gingerly, and seemed to revive. "Gentlemen, I have said what must be said in the 29th Bulletin, which is already in urgent dispatch to Paris. There are men of strong and there are men of feeble minds. It is whether we conquer ourselves that really matters." Napoleon wasn't quite sure whether he believed this last or not, and found himself crossing the Beresina once again. The ice floes cracked and creaked beneath the bridges. "All the world knows how such things are managed when I am in the field. I couldn't help that the river should have risen so with the rain and snow. It was of no consequence when we advanced. But still, I am the Emperor Napoleon!" The Emperor laughed. "And I am married to a Habsburg Princess!" The Emperor laughed some more, and the Abbé and the two ministers laughed with him. Such is the power of Emperors.

"In Russia, I could not help it freezing" the Emperor continued. "They told me every morning that I had lost 10,000 horses during the night - Well, farewell to them! Our Norman horses are less hardy than the Russians - they sink under ten degrees of cold below zero. It is the same with the men. There is but a short step from the sublime to the ridiculous. Look at the Bavarians. There is not one left. Perhaps it may be said that I stopped too long at Moscow; that may be true, but the weather was fine - the winter came on prematurely - besides, I expected peace. I sent Lauriston to treat for peace! I thought of going to St. Petersburg, and I had time enough to have done so. Bah! Well, we will make head at Vilnius. Ney is left there. Ha, ha, ha! It is a great political game, gentlemen. Nothing venture, nothing win after all."

"Quite so" said the Abbé. The two Polish ministers nodded uneasily. It seemed to them the venture was more theirs than Napoleon's. If the defeat of the Grande Armée was as they began to suspect, they would await the advance of the Cossacks into the Grand Duchy, whilst the guarantor of both their dreams and their forthcoming disaster would most certainly depart. "It is but a small step from the sublime to the ridiculous" observed Napoleon once again. The two ministers coughed in alarmed agreement, the step seeming far too small for comfort.

Napoleon clapped his hands in front of the dying fire. "The Russians have shown great character. Their Emperor is beloved by his people - they have clouds of Cossacks. The peasants of the crown love their government. The nobility are all mounted on horseback. I made regular war on Alexander, but who could have expected the burning of Moscow?" The burning of Moscow! The hairs on the heads of the three listeners stood rigid at the very thought. What scale of calamity was this? "Aye, gentlemen". Even Napoleon seemed to acknowledge the dark destructions of bloody and hellish war that had been waged. How would it be if it were Paris that so burned? The Emperor's voice lowered to a penetrating, almost defensive, whisper. "Now they would lay it on us, but it was Rostopchin that did it. That sacrifice would have done honour to ancient Rome."

The fire went out. The Abbé and the two ministers stood in frozen despair as the Emperor paced ever faster up and down the room, desperate himself to keep warm, but still more desperate to find some brilliant manoeuvre that would yet engineer his and the destroyed Grande Armée's recovery. He returned to his project of raising 10,000 Polish swordsmen. The ministers explained the difficulties in conscripting such a number. Who would feed them? And where would the horses come from? The Polish stock was much diminished by the war already. Napoleon continued to walk, faster and faster, up and down, backwards and forwards across the room, seemingly oblivious to the reservations to his new strategy so raised. "I must have them" he said. At last, as if exhausted, and nothing new concluded, his monologue ended, terminated finally by another utterance of the aphorism he had just rendered immortal concerning the close proximity of the ridiculous to the sublime. When finally the Emperor stopped pacing up and down, he discovered his three companions had their heads pointing firmly down towards the floor.

Eventually, the Abbé de Pradt inquired whether Napoleon intended to make way to Paris through Silesia. "Ha! Prussia" said the Emperor. "Do you think it no longer safe for me to travel through that kingdom?" The Ambassador lied, and observed he'd meant no such thing. "It's not safe for me anywhere outside the Tuileries" replied Napoleon. "There are rogues and opportunists everywhere." The burning of Moscow, the passage of the Beresina and the conspiracy of Malet all flamed at once to full fruition in his mind's eye. He raged within, his stomach sickened him once more, the flames grew higher and higher. "Is it my fault I am cast as the dictator of the world?" he screamed.

Caulaincourt re-entered the room, and seemed to have a calming effect on all present. The Duke of Vicenza's sledge was ready once more to depart. The Emperor immediately took on the Duke's identity again, as if relieved to be freed from himself. Meanwhile, Caulaincourt took a swig of brandy before resuming the role of his own valet, that saguine breed to whom no man is a hero, as the Abbé could not at this juncture avoid reflecting. Napoleon broke briefly from his disguise to cut short the respectful wishes of all present for the preservation of his health, adding finally "I could not be in better health were the very devil in me." The two ministers were still anxious to raise the matter of Polish defence against the imminent Cossacks, but Napoleon would brook no word of it. Caulaincourt coughed. He waited by the door impatient to escape, and the pretend Duke of Vicenza seemed in no mind to delay him. Duke and valet thus exited, the door was closed, and the horses sprung forward, nearly overturning the sledge as it crossed the courtyard and sped through the gate. And so the dictator of the world disappeared into the darkness.

The sledge sled on, making good progress for the addition of fresh horses, or rather horses and ponies, Caulaincourt having been unable to procure sufficient horses alone during the brief stop in the Grand Duchy. There were two horses and a pony on the right, one horse and two ponies on the left. The average stride on the left being thus shorter than on the right, the postillion had to frequently compensate the equine team's direction to the right in order to keep them on a straight path. Caulaincourt much admired the easy skill with which this was affected. Napoleon didn't notice.

Caulaincourt hadn't shaven for five days. He felt uncomfortable bearded, but remarked to himself that at least it helped fend off the cold from his face. His was a woolly, wholesome growth, thick with hoar-frost, yet warming nonetheless. Caulaincourt noticed that the Emperor was protected by no such abundance. For such an awesome specimen of heroic manhood, his beard was but light. Under Napoleon's chin was only a fine downy growth, and his cheeks lacked even that. So exposed to the elements, they were rosy red, almost like those of an over-aged cherub. Napoleon had to rub his cheeks for warmth with his gloved hands, whilst Caulaincourt's could remain firmly clasped in his lap throughout. The cold inside the sledge was so intense that the traveller's breath froze on their eyebrows and formed icicles beneath their noses. The clothwork of the upholstery more properly resembled metallic sheets of ice. Caulaincourt was desperate for sleep, but to sleep in such frozen circumstances for more than half an hour was to risk death, and the Emperor so obviously preoccupied with matters of state, Caulaincourt didn't trust to be woken in time from any slumbers he might take to, however welcome they might be. He thus resolved to stay awake until Paris.

The Emperor dozed off.

He was in Notre Dame. The gargoyles looked down on him, chanting mournfully. This is a prayer for the souls of the departed, for all the young men who've died before they'd even started, for all the mothers of France weeping broken hearted, this is a prayer for the souls of the departed. *The souls came in a multitude from the altar, rising upwards towards the vaulted cathedral ceiling, which miraculously parted, allowing their journey to continue ever upwards, towards the Heavens.* This is a prayer for the souls of the departed. *Josephine was there too, holding in her arms a dead baby, which for one horrifying moment looked to Napoleon like the King of Rome. "This is for our love" she said, beckoning him to hold it. The Emperor declined, and, asking of its sex, and was relieved to hear it was a girl. Josephine burst into tears, and was led away arm in arm by a naked woman come to tend her grief. As the naked woman turned towards him, Napoleon recognised her for the Empress Marie-Louise. She was wearing a tiara and nothing more. Her Emperor couldn't help noticing the fullness of her breasts, or the inviting swing and swagger of her backside. She had been taking lessons from Josephine after all. The gargoyles turned on him, as if aware of his innermost thoughts.* This is a prayer for the souls of the departed, for all the young men who died before they'd even started. *More and more dead souls, a seeming infinitude, came up from the altar, with faces that seemed to Napoleon to be outside the spheres of retribution or forgiveness, knowing only an untroubled beatitude he had never seen before. The vaulted ceiling continued to open wider and wider, letting in an unearthly light that beckoned on the spirits ever skywards.* For all the mothers of France weeping broken hearted, this is a prayer for the souls of the departed, *sang the gargoyles, louder and louder, but with a perfect pitch in seeming contradiction of their distorted features.*

The Emperor woke up. Caulaincourt shivered, a sudden shaft of cold running down his back as if he was sitting next to the devil himself. The Emperor told Caulaincourt to stop singing. Caulaincourt said he hadn't been singing anything. The sledge came abruptly to a halt. They were at the Prussian border.
"Who is it?" said the guard.

"The Duke of Vicenza and his valet", said Caulaincourt, at once dismounting.

"Where are you going?"

"To Dresden."

"What for?"

"It is private business."

This was the moment Caulaincourt had been dreading. Had news yet reached the border that Napoleon had left the Grande Armée? And if so, had news travelled also of the parlous state of the Grande Armée itself? If so, the Prussian king could have already switched allegiances, and issued the necessary warrants for his Emperor's arrest. Luckily it was dark, but his travelling companion retained the most famous visage in Europe. The guard walked around the sledge.

The Emperor-as-fugitive thought the real Duke of Vicenza. "Has he luck?" The Emperor always asked that to assess a man's practical value. And now, as Caulaincourt nervously observed, it applied to him. Would the guard open the door, or would he not? If he did, would the Emperor be recognised, or would he not? Or would he give himself away with his imperial presence? All these speculations seemed but small ways of raising the larger question. *Was Russia a temporary set back or the beginning of the end?* The guard rubbed on the window glass of the sledge, warming the frost with his elbow to partially dislodge it. "Have I luck?" Napoleon thought to himself from inside. He had wrapped his head, all but his nostrils and forehead, in furs, and was feigning sleep. "Have I the luck?" The guard peered inside. "Have I still the luck?" For the first time since he was an *étoile* of the military school at Paris, Napoleon Bonaparte, Emperor of the French, found himself questioning his *own sense of destiny*!

"He could die like that", said the guard.

"He's not been asleep long", replied Caulaincourt. "And he's well wrapped up."

"More than we are."

The guard stamped his feet on the snowy ground.

"Sorry?" said Caulaincourt, noticing he had already started to copy the guard's movements without realising it. The two of them compounded the snow in two pairs of footprints some two yards apart.

"He's got half your furs wrapped round him, hasn't he?" said the guard.

"I gave them to him", said Caulaincourt.

"Dukes, kings and emperors. They're all the bleedin' same."

"I've only ever served one."

"What's in the trunks?" said guard.

"Personal effects."

"Personal what? I could keep you here all night."

"Wouldn't you rather be in your hut?"

"It's my duty to stop you. I've got my orders."

Caulaincourt had come to the conclusion that bribery was unlikely to work with this man, and yet was aware their meeting must move on. But just what did the guard want? The two of them were still stamping their feet up and down whilst moving nowhere. At length the guard moved back towards the partially defrosted window, which was already refreezing up.

"So what does your Duke want with Dresden then?"

"It's private. Very private."

"How very?"

The guard rubbed ferociously with his elbow on the window glass, making a circular viewing space some nine or ten inches in diameter. He peered in, beadily. The Emperor coughed involuntarily, and then moved his head towards the area of the window through which the guard looked in, as if moving in his sleep. The idea had been to block the guard's view as if innocently, but the movement seemed only to make the Prussian prosecutor more suspicious.

"I could ask him myself you know", said the guard, fixing his hand on the sledge door handle.

"He'd say the same thing as me, only he'd be much ruder", replied Caulaincourt.

Napoleon suddenly became aware he still had the Imperial seal on his finger. He thought of taking it off, but was aware the guard still had one eye fixed on the window. And besides, to take off the seal he would have to take off his gloves first, which, even allowing for such a somnambulant practice, would appear very strange in such cold weather, be he asleep or waking. And then, he suspected his digits to be so swollen with the cold that any removal would prove prolonged and problematic of itself. With the acute wisdom of a born leader, Napoleon left the Imperial seal where it was. He would yet need it. The guard turned the door handle. Both the real and the pretend Duke of Vicenza held their breath. The guard pulled the door towards him. It stuck. It had frozen solid.

"Just as well", said Caulaincourt. "You wake up the Duke of Vicenza at your peril."

"Look. You can't just wander around Europe without a bye or a leave you know", said the guard, by now indignant. "Ever since that Napoleon marched on Russia, it's been the same. People and persons of all sorts coming and going across the border like it was nobody's business but their own."

Caulaincourt decided to risk naked innocence. "Have you any news of the Grande Armée?"

"I don't know anything. And I don't care. All I care about is my border. Now, for the last time, I want to know exactly where you and your Duke are going, who you're going to see, and why."

The guard stamped his feet up and down again, compounding two new patches of snow in the vain effort to keep warm. Caulaincourt again found himself following suit, and, observing the tedium of this repetition, decided at once to take the initiative. He would speak to this truculent fellow as a knowing equal. He would confide in him, man to man. Caulaincourt took the guard to one side, placing his arm around his obstructer's shoulder as if in lasting friendship.

"Between you and me, it's a woman."

"What sort of a woman?"

"A very beautiful woman, who is quite smitten with the good Duke, as he is with her. Our trunks are full of presents for her."

"If it's a woman", said the guard, "then why the big secret? There are lots of women."

"This is a woman the Duchess of Vicenza doesn't know about."

"OOOOOOhhhhhh!"

"Now you see the delicacy?"

"Of course."

Caulaincourt congratulated himself. At the suggestion of adultery, the guard had quite changed his tune. An adulterer himself, doubtless. The guard smiled.

"Last summer I found my wife in a haystack with my brother. I went straight down to the asylum and found a lunatic to run them both through. And then I cried in church at the funeral with the best of them."

At this the guard laughed heartily, and slapped Caulaincourt hard on the back. Caulaincourt cursed his luck. He'd played the wrong tactic after all! Here was a fellow so morally indignant he was likely to have both himself and the Emperor arrested as conspirator to illicit fornication and committer of the very act respectively.

"What d'you think of that then? What d'you think of that?" rejoiced the guard.

"Very... Forthright", mused Caulaincourt.

"Nobody makes a fool out of me."

"Clearly."

"Got any drink?" said the guard with great purpose.

"Only a little vodka" said Caulaincourt.
"Let's have it then."
"The door's frozen up."
"Not the one you got out of."
"It's very rough."
"The rougher the better."

Caulaincourt had no choice but to oblige, albeit with great regret. The vodka he had taken from the Hôtel d'Angleterre was the only thing he had to keep his innards warm. He reached inside the sledge, and fumbled beneath the seating. His predicament was doubly troublesome, since he had told not even the Emperor that the vodka was there.

"What's that?" whispered Napoleon.
"A passport."

Caulaincourt duly handed over the vodka to its wrongful owner.

"Can we go now?"
"You must have some food as well."
"But we'll starve."
"D'you want to go, or don't you?"

Caulaincourt opened the unfrozen door once again, and reached back inside the sledge, fetching a half-ham and two somewhat frozen pieces of unleavened bread. As he was removing the ham, the gloved hand bearing the Imperial seal secured itself against his arm.

"I didn't know about the vodka, but I know about the ham. And I'm hungry" whispered Napoleon.
"So's the guard."

Caulaincourt looked at his Emperor. His Emperor looked at the ham.

"I think the ham will do it Your Majesty."
"It better", said Napoleon, "or I'll be out there myself."

This last was exactly what Caulaincourt dreaded. An indignant Emperor-pretending-not-to-be-an-Emperor railing at an obstreperous guard who was almost bound to recognise him if only because never in his life would such a small man have risen to such a great height before him. And the scene would be even worse if laced with alcohol! Caulaincourt walked with the ham to the already vodka drinking Prussian, and handed it over.

"I hope it's not off", he said.

"Not very likely in this weather is it?"

The guard took it, greedily.

"Can we go now?"

"Of course. And you can tell your Duke that I hope he catches the pox. Adulterers are the scum of the earth."

Caulaincourt climbed back into the sledge. The guard lifted the barrier. The postillion, silent throughout, cracked the horses and ponies forward, and the sledge slid on its way. The guard lowered the barrier, and retired into his hut for a night of inebriate denial of the cold.

Napoleon unwrapped the furs from his head.

"Is there no more vodka? My stomach is wretched."

"No Your Majesty."

"What did he say?"

"He said he hopes you catch the pox."

"You should have taken his name. I'd have had him punished when I restore my fortunes."

At this sign of Imperial determination, Caulaincourt reflected he should have been heartened, but instead he felt somewhat chilled. Did the Emperor know just how difficult it was going to be? And what would be the cost? Not another Russian campaign surely?

"The mistake I made Caulaincourt, is not the obvious one. It is not that I tried to accomplish in one campaigning season what should have taken two. It is that we failed to accomplish in six months what should in fact have taken merely four."

Caulaincourt confessed to being bemused. The Emperor proceeded to talk cheerfully of an imminent Polish revolution which would stop the Russians from crossing the Niemen, and so scare the Tsar Alexander he would treat for peace. "And even if he doesn't, Europe is so terrified of Alexander I will still find allies aplenty."

Caulaincourt decided upon direct contradiction.

"It is not Alexander they are terrified of Your Majesty. It is yourself. Europe fears your universal monarchy, your spreading family dynasty, the taxes your Empire imposes, and the levies you place on the youth through conscription. All this makes the hatred of you into a national force."

"It is but only so in reversal. When we are winning, I am adored" replied Napoleon. To this Caulaincourt did not reply.

Napoleon found some aniseed in his inner pockets, and sucked on it surreptitiously. He was about to continue his strategic monologue, when he noticed they were passing through Walewice. The Emperor was at once enthusiastic to stop. He wished to visit the chateau of his mistress Maria Walewska, who he was sure would provide them with succour of all kinds. And though yet still many miles from the King of Rome, he could see his other son Alexandre-Florian. Maria the Emperor knew to be devoted to him, and would be delighted.

"We could wash, and eat, and shave. And sleep" he said.

Caulaincourt doubted it was sleep that was most on Napoleon's mind, and chose to remind his Emperor of the urgency with which they must return to Paris. Quite apart from affairs of state, Marie-Louise would be frantic with worry.

"She will have worried for months", said the Emperor. "It makes no difference."

At length, Napoleon ordered the sledge to stop. There was then an argument, the Emperor wishing to make urgent haste to Walewice, Caulaincourt arguing any sojourn with the Countess Walewska was too pregnant with risk. The postillion sat immobilised, shivering to the sound of argumentative mumblings within, an extract of which ran as follows:

"Who's the Emperor in here?"

"Who's the Duke of Vicenza?"

Eventually, after much heated discussion, the party continued their journey to Dresden. The real Duke of Vicenza had won. The Emperor was, however, most offended by Caulaincourt's suggestion that his beloved Countess might betray him. He well knew that to women, power is the strongest of aphrodisiacs, and obviously, this made Napoleon alluring beyond all mere mortal measure. How little of women Caulaincourt understood! But somehow, as their journey continued, and night turned into an overcast and inhospitable morning, the thought of betrayal returned to Napoleon again and again like a homing pigeon. What did Caulaincourt think the chances were of the Prussians arresting them?

"Considerably higher if we involve the Countess Your Majesty."

"Yes, yes. But apart from her?"

"It is still the best part of a day to Dresden and Saxon safety. With each hour we must be sanguine."

Caulaincourt was aware of Napoleon's tendency to melancholy. He had probably sought the company of the Countess to cheer himself up. Caulaincourt tried to inject some humour into the proceedings.

"The Prussians wouldn't know what to do with us. They'd probably call a conference to avoid making a decision."

"And eventually I'd be handed over to the English. But then, I've always wanted to meet Wellington" Napoleon laughed.

"You could play chess together. You'd win."

"He'd cheat. The English would exhibit me in an iron cage in the middle of London, smear me with honey, and wait for me to be devoured by flies."

Caulaincourt laughed. "How fiendish."

"They'd do it to you too" Caulaincourt stopped laughing. So did Napoleon. For one who was used to striding continents as he pleased, the idea of captivity came abhorrent. "The English will never capture me", said the Emperor, darkly. Here he reflected was a fate worse than death itself.

At midnight on the 13th of December, the pair finally arrived in Dresden. Napoleon thought of the pomp that had surrounded his arrival in the Saxon capital only the previous May, but there were no dukes and duchesses, kings and queens or empresses and emperors for a reception committee this time. They were seeking the house of Monsieur de St. Aignan, the French minister, but had no written record of where it was, and so drove aimlessly around the streets until they found a lighted window. Caulaincourt called up, and a man in a nightcap put his head out of the window to ask them what they wanted. Caulaincourt explained they sought the French minister on urgent business, at which the man slammed his window shut. The Emperor said it would have been better to say they were seeking the King of Saxony direct, but Caulaincourt thought such grand ambitions too conspicuous. He was adamant the Duke of Vicenza would say no such thing.

By luck and chance, at three o'clock on the morning of the 14th of December they eventually found St. Aignan's residence, and after that diplomatist's astonishment had passed, they were entertained in seclusion with wine, cheese, sausage and pickles served directly by St. Aignan himself. The Emperor drank a great deal of wine, but the condition of his stomach still denied him the consumption of much food. He did, however, sit down to dictate several letters, which Caulaincourt dutifully transcribed. The most prominent of these documents was a letter to the Emperor of Austria. In it, the Emperor of the French assured his Imperial equal (he meant no such thing) that he had no plans to ferment Polish revolution or independence, and never have had. In short, he wished the Emperor Francis to consider his northern borders permanently secure, and added artfully that if they weren't, he had the Russian Tsar to blame, not his loyal son by marriage. He went on to say he was safe and well, as he prayed was the Emperor's daughter, his own wife, whom he was greatly looking forward to shortly seeing. He ended the letter by informing his father-in-law of his hope and confidence and of the army he would raise on the Niemen come the spring, with, he trusted, Austrian corps attached. The alliance of the French and the Austrian Emperors was, he felt sure, as cordial and as secured by natural justice as ever.

Napoleon then instructed St. Aignan to call the King of Saxony immediately. St. Aignan replied it was an ungodly hour to do any such thing. The Emperor said he was awake, and so why should the King of Saxony be asleep? The King of Saxony was duly summoned, and appeared most nervous. The 29th Bulletin had already reached him, and it was obvious to Caulaincourt that the King was astonished at Napoleon's change of fortune. Napoleon, however, was convinced the King was simply beside himself for being so singularly in the presence of so great a rearranger of the world.

"It is only the matter of Polish independence that can so distress you" said the Emperor. "But let me assure you of this. I will return within a few weeks, more powerful than ever, and then I shall ensure that the kingdom of Poland, for so long an old and cherished

Saxon dream, becomes yours at last. I will broke no argument on this point, as I have already informed the Austrians."

With this, the King of Saxony was dismissed, but not before he had promised many delicacies from the royal kitchens and wines from the cellars to accompany Napoleon on his continued journey in the morning. The sledge that had thus far traversed the Emperor would be of little use in the more mild country he and Caulaincourt had still to cross, and so the King's coach was commandeered with eight fresh horses, frisky beasts that much delighted the postillion. As yet, the coach was mounted on runners for the remains of the snow, but very soon they would go westwards by wheels on solid ground. From Dresden, real and pretend Dukes of Vicenza would travel with increased speed.

Over the next two days, they travelled through Leipzig and Auerstadt, through Erfurt and Frankfurt, finally crossing the Rhine at Mainz on the 16th of December 1812. The Emperor was within the natural boundaries of France once again! Here he was still the monarch absolute, undiminished by disaster, and he delighted in his new found freedom. He abandoned his incognito, restoring the title of Duke of Vicenza to its rightful owner, who was however chiefly gratified that the weather had grown warmer. The Emperor still wrapped himself up in furs, but he took off his gloves, and held up his Imperial seal to the light of the coach's window glass. It glistened, regally.

Caulaincourt, aware of his duty to posterity, started to consider an account of this most remarkable journey to be published as a journal, and so saw fit to question his Emperor on matters of strategy and statesmanship he felt remained unresolved.

"The French nation is the liberator of the world Caulaincourt!" exclaimed Napoleon. "Consider the revolution. We stand for the most sacred rights of peoples and nations, whereas the English only ever defend their self-assumed privileges."

"I see", said Caulaincourt. "And your thoughts on the Russian campaign?"

"We could have accomplished in four months what we failed to achieve in six. Consider this. I should have crossed the Niemen with an army of but 300,000. 600,000 was too large. With a smaller number I would have had greater flexibility, and my troops would have been mainly French alone. Our subject troops proved to have little stomach for the fight. I could then have pursued a narrow front at greater speed, ignoring the flanks save to invite the Prussians to defend Prussia, the Poles Poland and the Austrians Austria. I then declare the independence of Poland, guaranteeing Austria against any Polish threat from the north. That way, I could have crossed the Niemen in May to seize the Vitebsk-Orsha gap, moving so fast between the two Russian armies of Barclay and Bagration that they were prevented from ever joining. Then Smolensk would have been easy. You see?"

"I see Your Majesty. But you have still fought no battles."

"We should have moved the main supply bases up to Smolensk. Danzig and Königsburg were always too far back, and at Vitebsk and Minsk, we let vast stores fall into Russian hands. By basing our supplies at Smolensk, we could have defeated each Russian army in detail as Barclay and Bagration attempted to move up ahead or behind us."

"But what of the revolution?"

"Ah", said the Emperor. "The French are the liberators of the world! We should have gained the mass of the Russians on our side, by announcing the freedom of the serfs, throwing aristocracy and peasants against each other, and insuring ourselves against partisan retaliation. The partisans would have been on our side! With serf support and a smaller army, feeding the mass would have been much easier, and so we would have reached Moscow earlier, in August. I could then have treated for peace with the Tsar, informing him that if he didn't co-operate, I would send half the army to capture St. Petersburg, and the other half to overwhelm the Russian bases at Kaluga and Tula. The Tsar would have been left with two choices. To treat for peace on my terms, or to leave Russia without either of her capitals, without an army, without supplies and with the vast majority of the people, the serfs, on our side. Simple! My mistake was to forget the revolution Caulaincourt. And a Frenchman must never do that. The revolution is our greatest asset."

Caulaincourt couldn't help reflecting the Emperor was truly a Corsican, but let it pass. Napoleon suddenly felt drowsy, and strangely passive.

"It's a shame our will deserts us as we get older", he said at length. "I am forty three. Alexander the Great never had this problem. He was dead at thirty two."

Caulaincourt was staggered. Here was his Emperor, at one moment re-planning his most ambitious campaign, and at the next lamenting his declining powers!

"I was bored when I marched on Russia" said Napoleon. "And I still am. How far is it to Paris?"

"Forty eight hours more Your Majesty."

"I say thirty six."

Caulaincourt felt immediately relieved. The Emperor had clearly rediscovered his determination, and was impatient to be home. Some minor matters, however, yet delayed them. They had to stop several times to change from runners to wheels and back again, being consistently on wheels alone only from Verdun onwards. And just beyond Verdun, an axle breakage caused them to transfer to an open cabriolet. But this proved unreliable and rattlesome, and at Meaux they made their final change to a postmaster's post-chaise, a cumbersome carriage with two enormous wheels. Napoleon fell silent after his mental reviewing of the Russian campaign. Caulaincourt was too stimulated by the wonders of seeing his native countryside again to do anything other than look around him in wide-eyed amazement. Miraculous!

The Emperor fell asleep.

He was re-crossing the field of Borodino once again. There were lying on the field 80,000 dead soldiers, although Napoleon could not make out which were French and which Russian. All the uniforms seemed to be the same. Universally blood coloured.
"What did you expect?" said a dead soldier, rising one legged from the ground with the help of two others, one lacking an arm, the other an eye. "The same blood flows through all our veins."
The three dead soldiers beckoned the Emperor on. The Emperor followed. A dead horse, disembowelled but still chewing grass, fixed him in the eye, and winked.
"I haven't got a stomach left, but I still like the taste. Grass is wonderful. Don't you agree?"
The Emperor didn't know what to say. The horse continued.
"This isn't Borodino you know. This is the ghost of the revolution. How does it feel?"
The Emperor wasn't sure. A crowd started to gather around the horse. There were other horses, women, cattle, children, ponies, and soon, it would seem, eighty thousand men. Each of the dead was rising from the field, a multitude of walking-wounded afterlife, every single one of them broken and bloody, every single one of them defaced or deformed by the

violence they had done to each other in someone else's name.

"It was in your name", said a child, "that my parents were killed."

"I was raped seventeen times" said the woman.

"Who by?" said Napoleon.

"Can't you see that's not the point!" said a cow with both ears and one leg missing. "You made us walk all the way from the fields of France to Moscow", the cow continued. "What was wrong with the fields of France?"

"You don't understand", said the Emperor. "The Russians were threatening me. Besides, they wanted the war."

"You wanted the war", said another child, sitting astride a blind pony.

The black skies opened. A shaft of light lit the scene. The disembowelled horse came to the front of the still gathering crowd, each mortal soul of which stepped sideways to let him through. The crowd of the dead, it seemed, was a gathering throng which would gather forever. The horse continued chewing the cud, clearly about to say something of great import. As he swallowed, the cud fell from a gaping wound below the horse's neck back to the ground. But the horse continued to chew nonetheless. He winked at Napoleon again.

"It's the taste." And then the horse raised his neck, looked down on the Emperor, and disseminated his wisdom:

"What a pity it has been to see a mind so great as yours devoted to trivial things such as empires, great historic events, the thundering of cannons and of men. You believe in glory, in posterity, in Alexander and Caesar. Nations in turmoil and other trifles of time absorb all your attention. Why is it that you cannot see what really matters is something else entirely?"

"What is it?" said Napoleon.

"You either know or you don't know" said a chorus of dead soldiers. *"You can't be told."*

The Emperor was lost for words.

"What is it?" he said again.

"You either know or you don't know" said the entire company of dead men and horses and children and ponies and women and cattle in unison. *Everyone drew in closer to the Emperor in their midst.*

"Don't kill me", said Napoleon. "Please don't kill me!"

The Emperor was surrounded. The skies brightened, he was blinded by light. He closed his eyes in fear. And then, nothing. Tick, tick, tick. Nothing. Napoleon opened his eyes.

"Nothing has happened, and nothing is going to" said the horse.

The crowd stood, deathly silent. The Emperor fainted, but awakened again almost immediately, finding himself lying face upwards on the field of Borodino, starring at the sky. The sun shone brightly. The faces of the crowd peered blithely down on him. He noticed all the children were smiling, but couldn't think why. In fact, Napoleon Bonaparte, Emperor of the French, couldn't think anything at all. He was paralysed.

"I'm the emperor of the field I was born in" said a pony.

"I'm the empress of the village bar in Montaillou" said a woman.

"And I'm the emperor of the bakery at Smolensk" said a soldier.

"I'm the emperor of the village of Studenka."

"I'm the empress of the blacksmith's at Smorgoni."

The horse winked at Napoleon once again.

"We're all emperors and empresses here you know."

"I'm the empress of the world!" said a little girl, "I live everywhere."

"So do I" said a motherless foal.
"We all live everywhere."
"Emperors and empresses, every single one of us."
Napoleon could feel the ground collapse beneath him as he started falling straight down into Hell. He was scared to death, and too scared to admit it.

"Your Majesty!" Caulaincourt had great difficulty waking Napoleon from his slumbers. "Your Majesty!" The post-chaise had reached Paris, and was travelling up the Cours de Vincennes towards the Rue de Rivoli. As they passed the Hôtel de Ville, the Tuileries came fully into view. It was half-past eleven on the evening of the 18th of December 1812. The Emperor was home at last.

At so late an hour, Napoleon and Caulaincourt had difficulty in entering the Tuileries. The Empress had retired to her private apartment. Two muffled figures in furs entered the ante-chamber, and the shorter of them directed his course to the door of the Empress's sleeping chamber. Napoleon's thoughts returned to her fair innocent skin, and to the entry of the ancient Habsburgs. This time he could feel the rising in his loins. The lady in waiting hastened to throw herself between the seeming intruder and the entrance, but, recognising the Emperor, she shrieked out loud, and so alarmed Marie-Louise, who thus entered the room in her night-gown. The Empress looked with astonishment across the room at her Corsican conqueror, who, dishevelled and unshaven, could only stare back at her, dumbstruck. Marie-Louise had read the 29th Bulletin, and looked Napoleon up and down as if taking in his abrupt change of circumstance. Here stood her husband after all, whom she had previously presumed to be not so much a favourite of Fate, but rather Fate itself.

"It is I" said the Emperor, thinking once again of openly inhabiting his beloved dark-green uniform. "The Emperor. I'm still the Emperor. Still."

TELLING STORIES No.2

The Letter to the Immortal Beloved continues as follows:

(6 July, in the morning, contd.)

My journey was a fearful one and I did not arrive here until yesterday at four o'clock in the morning. As there were few horses the mail coach chose another route, but what a dreadful road it was; at the last stage but one I was warned not to travel by night; attempts were made to frighten me about the forest, but all this only spurred me onwards - but I was wrong. The coach must needs break down, of course, owing to the wretched road which had not been made up and was nothing but a bottomless mudded track. If I hadn't had two such postillions I should have been left stranded on the way - Esterházy travelling the other usual road with eight horses met with the same fate as did I with four - Yet I felt to a certain extent pleasure from my trials that I always feel when I have overcome some difficulty successfully - Now, let me turn quickly from things external to things internal. We shall surely see each other soon; and today also time fails me to tell you of the thoughts which during these last few days I have had touching my own life - If our hearts were always closely united, I would certainly have none of these. My heart overflows with a longing to tell you so many things - ah - there are moments when I find that speech amounts to nothing at all - Be cheerful - and be for ever my faithful, my only sweetheart, my all, as I am yours. The gods must send us the rest, whatever must and shall be our fate -

Your faithful

LUDWIG

What sort of a mood is Beethoven in? Like Esterházy, he's had a difficult journey. But Esterházy is hardly his chief concern. Beethoven's travelled by night, through darkening forests on dreadful roads. It's been a struggle to get where he's got to, but get there he must. *Fate* demands it. Beethoven's exhausted and yet he doesn't mention sleeping. He's exhausted and yet he's probably been up all night. The urge to write is clearly overpowering, despite the fact he can hardly think straight. His heart is pounding with excitement and expectation that "we shall surely see each other soon." And Beethoven's head is pounding too. Whatever the need to tell of the *external* story of his journey, perhaps to demonstrate to his Immortal Beloved the difficulties he has overcome simply to rendezvous with her, his *internal* stories and thoughts are much more important to him. His *internal* thoughts, stories and yes, his dreams too, are everything. Beethoven can hardly write in sentences - his letter is rapidly generating dashes by the score. Beethoven's heart is overflowing, spilling over with seemingly everything in the world he has ever wished to tell anyone. His heart is racing, his head is spinning. He can't go on with out sleep and rest, but he goes on without sleep and rest nonetheless.

Look at the original manuscript of the letter, first and last pages. The handwriting, barely legible at best, gets larger and less legible as the letter goes on. By the end of the letter, there is barely one word per line, and it's verging on illegible scribble. Except that it's everything more. Beethoven is tearing at the paper. The dashes are not dashes but searing and seething cries of anguish at separation and love at imminent reunion and *emotions-beyond-words* across the page. Beethoven here is on the edge of nowhere and on the brink of everything. It is well worth noting that in the original German, this is the only letter Beethoven ever wrote where he addresses a woman by the familiar German "Du" instead of the more formal "Sie." Beethoven is doing everything for the first time. He's romantically impassioned, but treading virgin ground.

Who is Esterházy? The only Esterházy Beethoven is known to have known is Prince Nikolaus Esterházy, who, in 1812 was the Austrian Ambassador to the Saxon court at Dresden. And in 1812 the 6th of July fell on a Monday. *So 1812 fits*. And in early July 1812, it's known that Beethoven was in Teplitz taking the waters on the advice of Dr. Malfatti, Teplitz being a renowned Bohemian spa town. And in early July 1812, it's known that Prince Esterházy was ordered to travel by Prince von Metternich from Vienna via Teplitz to Dresden with diplomatic dispatches. All of which means that the Letter to the Immortal Beloved could well have been written in Teplitz in 1812. Let's accept this as fact for now.

Crossing Out The Emperor

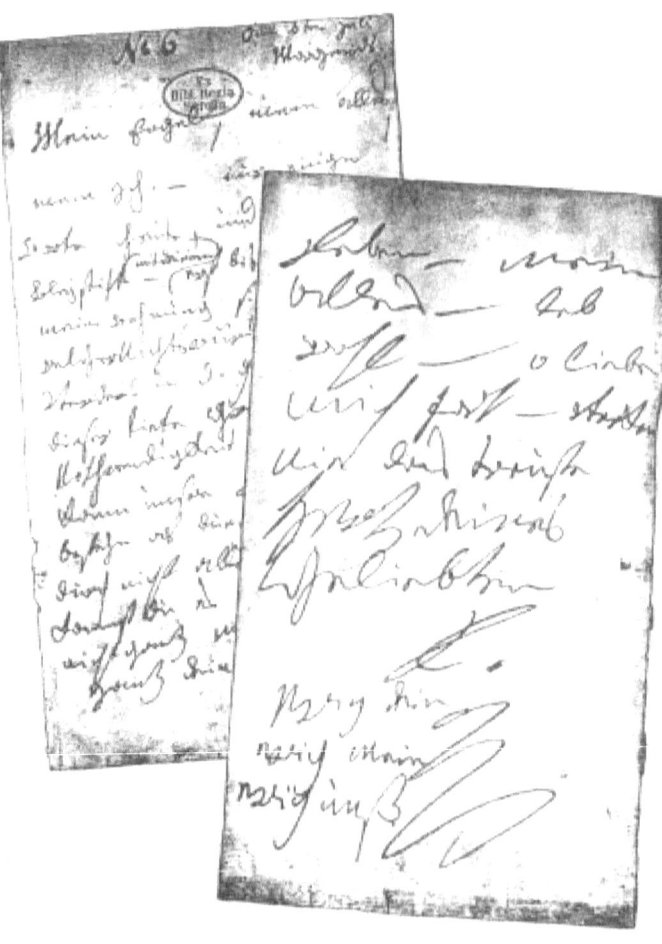

LETTER TO THE IMMORTAL BELOVED
first and last page

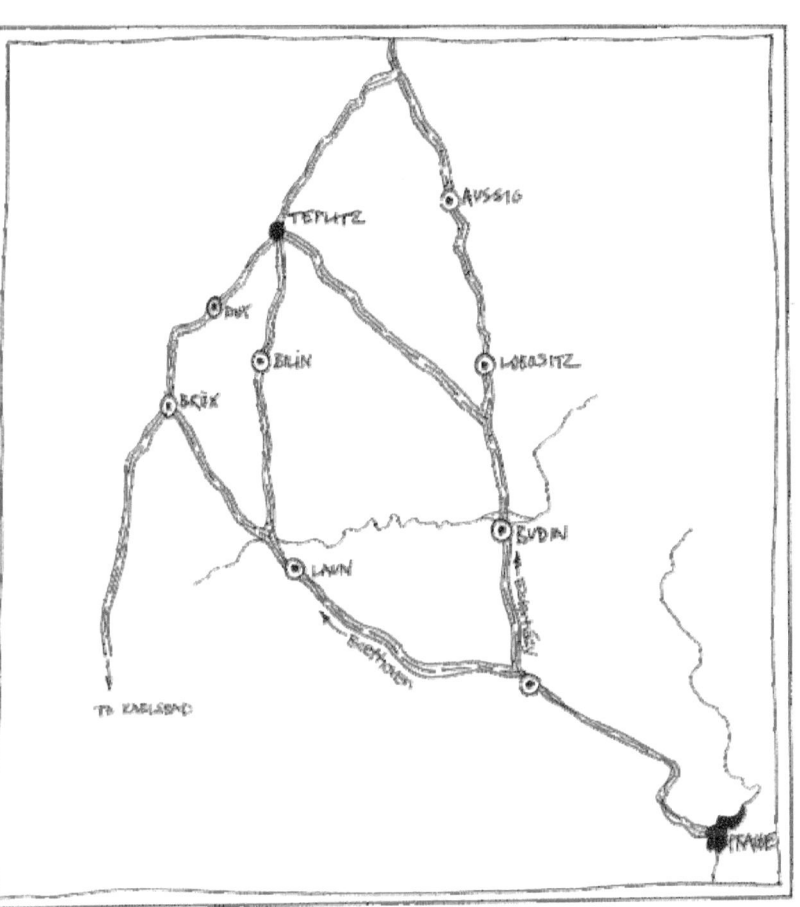

PROBABLE JOURNEYS OF BEETHOVEN AND ESTERHÁZY TO TEPLITZ, 1812

At the same time, Johann Wolfgang von Goethe was in the neighbouring spa town of Karlsbad, directly to the south. But Goethe wasn't there to take the waters, and he wasn't there seeking inspiration in the mountainous countryside either. Goethe was in Karlsbad as Privy Councillor to the Duke of Weimar, an advisory post to the Duke Goethe much enjoyed. And Goethe was in Karlsbad because he couldn't stand the rush of Teplitz.

Teplitz was normally quiet enough, but in July 1812 it was filling up with ambassadors, dignitaries and heads of state of all kinds. Indeed, the whole *charabanc* of dukes, princes, kings and the Austrian Emperor Francis who had greeted the Emperor Napoleon with such unctuous attentions at Dresden in June, was now rendezvous-ing anew to discuss *what they were supposed to do now?* They were all the allies of Napoleon largely under duress, and they all needed the healing waters of Teplitz as much as Beethoven had need of them himself. If Napoleon conquered Russia, he would be the undisputed master of the Continent from west to east, from south to north - and everyone considered Napoleon's success a foregone conclusion. The King of Saxony, the Prince of Courland, the Grand Duke of Würzburg, Goethe's master the Duke of Weimar, the Prussian Ambassador Baron von Humboldt, the Austrian government adviser Prince Karl Lichnowsky *(yes, the patron of Beethoven)* and the Emperor Francis of Austria himself all knew the score. And so, amidst this crowd of flat champagne and generally small beer royalty, did the civil servants, writers of "confidential memoranda" journalists, junior ministers, spies and woman of various degrees of charm, beauty and intellect that always accompany such a gathering, and in this case had accompanied it direct from their greeting of the Emperor Napoleon at Dresden. *The score was this.* If Napoleon conquered Russia, he would be the effective dictator of the world.

In Teplitz in 1812, no matter how long they bathed, the spa waters couldn't heal the assembled ruler's pain. The evening concerts and balls were tinged with a distinct air of diplomatic panic, of anxiety all permeating and unavoidable.

And in the midst of all this was Beethoven, in search of a quiet life for a change from the bustle and gossip of Vienna, only to find that virtually everyone important in Vienna had seemingly followed him to Teplitz! But whereas everyone else in Teplitz saw only a dark and dominated future, its possible Beethoven was contemplating exactly the opposite. He was contemplating union with his Immortal Beloved.

The retinue of the "Congress of Teplitz" stayed in Teplitz itself, or, like Goethe, in Karlsbad. The Karlsbad *Kurliste*, a voluntary register of visitors, states the following for June and July 1812. Present, amongst others, were:

Visitor
   Arrival

Elisabeth von der Recke
   June 7
Princess Moritz Leichtenstein with husband
   June 25
Baroness Dorothea Ertmann
   June 25
Antonie Brentano, with husband and child
   July 5

So, if we accept that Beethoven wrote his letter in Teplitz on Monday, the 6th of July 1812, then the Immortal Beloved can only be one of these four women. Yes? *Yes*. And let's accept the fairly universal consensus that Elise von der Recke and the Princess Leichtenstein aren't serious contenders. And I'm going to discount Dorothea von Ertmann, because whilst George Marek suggests her, even he admits he's not convinced. So we're left with Antonie Brentano, with husband and child. Here's Antonie's story.

Secretly, they rendezvous-ed in Prague. She had said everything he thought he'd never hear from a woman. He'd been rejected by peasant girls for peasant boys and by aristocrats aplenty for aristocrats. Magdalena Willman had sung his songs but concluded he was "ugly and half crazy." But to Antonie he was different. "You are everything" she said, "my whole life and all my dreams combined." Beethoven didn't know what to do. Every previous fault was suddenly a virtue. His tumult was inspiration, his unworldly habit of not listening to people simply proof of a divine creed. And he certainly listened to Antonie. Throughout the previous months he had found seeing her almost unbearable, yet somehow go on seeing her he had. His earlier interest in Bettina Brentano was but nothing in comparison to meeting her sister-in-law. Bettina had charmed and flirted, and been considerably miffed to be ousted by her sister-in-law in the first place, but Bettina also knew how to look after herself, and besides, she'd recently married Achim von Arnim. For six months, Beethoven had walked twice a week to Antonie's house, his feet almost floating on the pavement. For six months, Beethoven had been angry no longer. Instead he felt impetuous and yet kind, thoughtful and yet acutely aware of the necessity of quick action. "Ludwig", intervened Antonie, as they sat together in a cafe. "Are you listening to me?" She spoke not loudly but with great clarity and purpose. Beethoven marvelled that he could hear her without difficulty. "Yes, of course" he replied, "but I am also thinking of what we must do." In Prague, they were on their way somewhere, but uncertain as yet just where. The waiter asked them to order. Antonie ordered iced coffee for both of them. Beethoven wanted wine, but thought the better of it. This was a time for clear heads. What were they to do now? They both knew they would have to leave Vienna, perhaps for years to come, but surely with time the scandal would pass. And one thing Antonie knew for sure. She could never go back to Frankfurt. Antonie's days with Franz were over forever, her life with Beethoven just beginning. Her life with Beethoven and her daughter Maxe's too.

Maxe was ten, and busy playing with the napkins. Antonie and Beethoven felt it safer to whisper anyway, but with Maxe with them too, it was essential. Maxe must not, in her innocence, breathe a word to Franz, else she too would be lost. Antonie had married Franz Brentano, a banker and bourgeois fifteen years her senior, at her father's behest on July 23rd 1798. Antonie's father being none other than the noted Austrian statesman, scholar and art connoisseur Johann Melchior Edler von Birkenstock, the marriage was a very grand affair, and one at first most pleasing to all concerned. Franz, already building his bank in mercantile Frankfurt, was looking for an aristocratic wife to secure connections in Vienna. He wished to forge alliances between the north and the south speaking Germanic lands. Von Birkenstock, aware that the pace of development in the north was outstripping that in the south, wished the union success for the same reasons as Franz, but from the opposite perspective. And the young Antonie was the perfect symbol for such a plan, with her unblemished upbringing in an Ursuline convent at Pressburg and her impeccable manners. And moreover, she was pretty too. Her nose was perhaps a shade too long, but its fine boning had elegance, and her eyes shone brightly. Her curled hair framed her face with piquant charm, the effects on men of which its owner as yet barely understood. Antonie had "obediently yielded" to her father's wishes not knowing what else to do. And besides, Herr Brentano seemed kind enough. By 1806, Antonie had born five children, all but the first of which had survived. To all the world Franz and Antonie had everything, including an ostentatious mansion by the River Main. But all was not as it seemed. Franz was a naturally considerate man, and Antonie quickly developed deep affection for him, but of love there was none. And Frankfurt came to depress her utterly. She found her new home wholly strange and wept cold tears in solitude. In Frankfurt there was none of the art and gossip of Vienna, few or no visiting princes or princesses or counts and countesses to enliven the social calendar, and hardly any theatre or music worth speaking of. There were only money men by the score, and money is what money men speak of. Antonie came to regard it all as very vulgar. One never spoke of money in Vienna, one simply possessed it. But she understood her situation nonetheless. Franz worked at his bank all hours because he did not possess as much money as he wished to have. And neither, for that matter, did he yet possess as much money as he and Antonie stood to inherit through her father. Perhaps, thought Antonie, when Franz was satisfied, their lives would change. Perhaps they could move elsewhere, to an old and more cultured city such as Prague or to Berlin, or even back to Vienna itself! Oh, blessed thought, but no! In time, Antonie came to realise that Franz's appetite for money was insatiable, the driving appetite of all. For Franz, Frankfurt would always be perfect. Antonie took to calling it Franz-furt. She sighed and reflected often that she couldn't decide whether she didn't understand the bourgeois mind, or whether she simply despised it. Franz, the bourgeois paterfamilias, wished desperately to make Antonie happy, but ultimately, he simply didn't know how. Money did nothing to impress Johann von

Birkenstock's daughter. Antonie became irritable and had constant headaches. She rouged her face in a parody of the bourgeois Frau Franz half desired her to be. Franz thought she looked radiant. Antonie only laughed. Gradually, the light was losing its shine in her eyes. A deathly silence reigned within her soul.

And then a sad but welcome relief! In 1809, Antonie received news of her father's death, and she took at once the opportunity to move back to Vienna to settle the affairs of the estate. Quite apart from the von Birkenstock house itself, there were art treasures and manuscripts to deposit and auction to various museums and private collectors of all kinds. Although in mourning, Antonie delighted in Vienna's insouciance and artfulness once again, and it was with joy she came to share society gossip with the irrepressible Bettina, and the three von Brunsvik sisters Therese, Josephine and Charlotte. Through them she soon came to meet Luigi van Beethoven, by now Vienna's most sought after piano virtuoso and composer. In Frankfurt she had heard much of him, but he had never travelled there to play. In Frankfurt Antonie had not even been easily able to secure the score of a piece by now so famous as the Moonlight Sonata. Soon enough, Antonie approached Beethoven for lessons in piano composition, to which the composer responded eagerly. There was immediately something about her sad diminished eyes and graceful yet mourning profile that attracted him. Her curled hair framed her face as if half disguising her own inner sorrow. Beethoven could see Antonie was unhappy, and sought to unlock the cause. They were soon in love.

And so it came to pass that Ludwig van Beethoven and Antonie Brentano sat together in a cafe in Prague on the 4th July 1812, sure enough of their intentions, but with the plan as yet half-hatched. They talked of freedom. For the first time in many years Ludwig could hear his own voice without difficulty. Antonie's eyes shone deeper than the brightest waters of the deepest wells in Heaven. Beethoven was to go on to Teplitz, claiming need of rest. Antonie, with Franz and Maxe, was to go to Karlsbad, claiming need of a cure for her headaches. Antonie wrote down her address on a piece of paper with a pencil, and gave both to Beethoven. She was to stay at the White Swan. "Keep the pencil" she said, "it is something of me with you." But what after Teplitz and Karlsbad? How would they meet up again, and where would they go? As Beethoven sat in his lodgings at The Oak in Teplitz at the end of his dreadful journey the next day, there was still much that worried him. Could he, a bachelor by habit if not by intention, come at the age of forty two to give himself up to a new family life? He was certain of his love for both Antonie and Maxe, but would Antonie herself be happy? She was proposing to give up her entire inheritance! If she left Franz as she intended, he would automatically take claim to all. Money problems were nothing new to Beethoven, but he knew they would be utterly new to Antonie. And her naive insistence that after Franz, money was something she never wished to speak of again worried him greatly. Money, he pondered, is spoken of much more frequently by those without it than by those with it. And then there were the other children. Did Antonie really propose to leave three of them behind? Beethoven knew well enough that the support of four children was utterly beyond him financially, and he knew also that if Antonie left Franz, he had first claim by law to all four of the children anyway, but even so! Antonie saw Beethoven as "natural, simple and wise, with pure intentions" but was that enough? Beethoven adored Maxe, but how would Maxe cope with being separated from her brothers and sister? And what agony would Thomas and Christophe and Fanny go through themselves? Perhaps the boys would be stoical, but Fanny, in Heaven's name, was only six! And would Franz invoke the law to claim Maxe back as his own too? How would Antonie cope with that? Beethoven had been out walking and all these thoughts constantly returned to his mind. He had returned to find a letter from the great Goethe proposing the two men meet. There was no higher honour than to meet such a one as Goethe, but frankly, Beethoven didn't care. He opened the window, and peered out into the evening, south over the mountains towards Karlsbad itself. His faith returned to him. Their love was true, as yet unconsummated but already complete. It was as if every thought of Antonie's came directly to him on the evening breeze. He sat down to write once again. He took out Antonie's pencil and held it lovingly, still confused himself, but strangely confident.

Evening, Monday, 6 July

You are suffering, my dearest creature - only now have I learned that letters must be posted very early in the morning on Mondays - Thursdays - the only days on which the mail coach goes from here to K. - You are suffering - Ah, wherever I am, there you are also - I will arrange it with you and me that I can live with you. What a life!!!! Thus!!!! Without you - pursued by the goodness of mankind hither and thither - which I as little want to deserve as I deserve it - Humility of man towards man - it pains me - and when I consider myself in relation to the universe, what am I and what is He - whom we call the greatest - and yet - herein lies the divine in man - I weep when I reflect that you will probably not receive the first report from me until Saturday - Much as you love me - I love you more - But do not ever conceal yourself from me - good night - As I am taking the baths I must go to bed - Oh God - so near! So far! Is not our love truly a heavenly structure, and also as firm as the vault of Heaven? –

One thing was certain. Antonie would refuse to go back to Frankfurt. She had managed to remain three years in Vienna whilst tending to matters of estate, but Franz was becoming impatient. Three years to tidy up the life of a dead father was long enough. Franz was a practical man, and he frequently swore blind that left to him, everything could have been settled within six months. Antonie would refuse to go back to Franz-furt, of that Beethoven was sure. The inexorable logic of this alone drove his passion onwards. Antonie wished to be his. He was more important to her than all a banker's money in the world could ever be. There was a knock at the door. Could it be her? Beethoven knew she was planning only to leave Franz the most cursory of notes, but perhaps she had done this already, and now stood outside, married still yet free, un-rouged and freshly beautiful anew. Beethoven opened the door. It was Goethe. "Herr van Beethoven, I am Goethe" he said. "I know" said Beethoven. Goethe stood at once tall, erect and imperious. He was dressed casually, yet still wore the badge of Privy Councillor to the Duke of Weimar. "Your Excellency, your Highness, your Honour. I am honoured" Beethoven added quickly. "I gather we have shared a correspondence with Bettina Brentano" said Goethe. "Yes", said Beethoven. Goethe clearly expected to be invited in, but Beethoven thought it better if they walked out. If he allowed Goethe into his lodgings, he would have to conceal his letter for one. And in his desire for secret union, Beethoven was convinced no other but Antonie must have knowledge of it. Besides, he had drunk all the wine.

The two artists were no sooner out in the street than Goethe espied the Emperor Francis of Austria and full entourage coming direct towards them. Goethe immediately stopped to bow. Beethoven walked straight on. Goethe was appalled. Beethoven pretended not to notice. "Don't you know who that was?" asked Goethe. "Of course I do" replied Beethoven. "Then why did you not bow?" "I have long perfected the habit of appearing oblivious to such things as rank and position your Highness. I find it is easier that way. And besides, amongst them was Prince von Metternich, whom I loathe..." Goethe stopped Beethoven to listen to the singing of an evening sparrow. The bird could not be seen, but Goethe was certain of its location amongst the roof tops. Beethoven swore he could hear nothing. "A man should listen to a bird's song or read a beautiful poem at least once a day" said Goethe. Beethoven walked on, and realising he hadn't eaten for a full three days, asked where Goethe intended them to eat. Goethe said he wasn't hungry, having been offered a buffet at several diplomatic functions during the day. Beethoven grew impatient. Goethe decided to change the subject. "What an effect this man Napoleon has had on us all" he said. "Yes" said Beethoven. "I met him once", continued Goethe. "It was at the Conference of Erfurt. And Napoleon sought me out. Can you believe that? Napoleon Bonaparte sought me out!" "You sought me out" said Beethoven. "I can believe anything. But I do not envy you. There was a time when I would very much liked to have met this Napoleon myself, but I would not like to now." Goethe didn't believe this for a moment, and was convinced Beethoven was jealous. Beethoven was convinced Goethe was convinced Beethoven was jealous, and was furious. "I have better things to do with my time than reminisce on meetings with the famous Herr Goethe" said Beethoven. "I am in love." "But an artist like you can never marry, surely?" said Goethe. "She is already married." "Oh, you mean you are having an affair" enthused Goethe. "Well, good for you! I presume the lady is one of your patrons as well." "That's not what I meant at all" said Beethoven, by now wishing no further truck with anything. "I am hungry, and you are not. Perhaps we could arrange to meet another time." "Yes of course" said Goethe, rather shocked. It was the first time anyone had expressed exasperation at meeting him in many, many years. This Beethoven was certainly the uncouth fellow everyone had led him to believe! "But one last thing. Tell me Herr van Beethoven, do you work best in the mornings, the afternoons or the evenings? I myself find the hours after the dawn the most convivial." Beethoven looked at Goethe shocked and disappointed. An amateur! "I work all the time Herr Goethe. Good evening."

Beethoven went straight back to his lodgings, forgetting to eat despite his hunger, which quickly passed and turned into a kind of light headed, highly unstable, and yet deeply invigorating energy. The night was cool, but Beethoven found himself sweating in abundance. He was still not sure of his course of action. The question of finding a new city in which to earn his living came to preoccupy him. Prague did not appeal to him, its significance in matters musical having constantly diminished since the Habsburg monarchs had left it for Vienna several centuries before. And surely there was no answer to be found with a minor Bonaparte at the court of Westphalia! To Antonie at least, it would simply appear an inferior Vienna. But then, even Westphalia would be better than the living death of Franz-furt. He had forgotten Antonie's surety of purpose! If they could only grip their faith firmly in their joining hands, they would yet be free. Free to love and free to live anew. Perhaps they could have children themselves, which might ease Antonie's pain of having only Maxe beside her. Beethoven still couldn't sleep and the night was long in passing. He tossed and turned, and found himself speaking direct to Antonie, so near and yet still a spa town and a mountain range away. He wanted her, truly, deeply, madly. He wanted to taste her, to go between her, to know fully and be surrounded by her scent. For the first time in his life, Ludwig van Beethoven had feelings way beyond those which any music he might compose could possibly express! Ludwig van Beethoven was smitten and swimming in a sea of anticipated union. He was up before the dawn, and, after washing, returned to the bed in which he had thought of Antonie all night to write to her anew. The first rays of the sun found their way into the room. Beethoven was still resolving contradictions, and yet further resolved to be united in Antonie's arms, at whatever cost. The landlady brought him breakfast, and fresh news of the postal service. As finally and ravenously he ate, Beethoven was spurred on further. He must have her:

Good morning, on 7 July

Though still in bed, my thoughts go out to you, my Immortal Beloved, now and then joyfully, then sadly, waiting to learn whether or not fate will hear us - I can live only wholly with you or not at all - Yes, I am resolved to wander so long away from you until I can fly to your arms and say that I am really at home with you, and can send my soul enwrapped in you into the land of spirits - Yes, unhappily it must be so - You will be the more contained since you know my fidelity to you. No one else can ever possess my heart - never - never - Oh God, why must one be parted from one whom one so loves. And yet my life in V is now a wretched life - Your love makes me at once the happiest and the unhappiest of men - At my age I need a steady, quiet life - can that be so in our connection? My angel, I have just been told that the mail-coach goes every day - therefore I must close at once so that you may receive the I at once. - Be calm, only by a calm consideration of our existence can we achieve our purpose to live together - Be calm - love me - today - yesterday - what tearful longings for you - you - you - my life - my all - farewell. - Oh continue to love me - never misjudge the most faithful heart of your beloved

(?)L/B/LB(?)

ever thine
ever mine
ever ours

With this, Beethoven got up out of bed, and walked at great pace straight down to the postal box. His mind was made up, his concerns and contradictions resolved, his new future with Antonie as certain as the very ground on which he paced. Only the worry that Franz himself, with Antonie in Karlsbad, might see the letter concerned him. But Antonie was surely clever enough to insure against that! And besides, what if Franz did read it? He would read only of what he would find out soon enough. Antonie was leaving him forever.

The next few days passed slowly. Antonie was an ever present absence, Beethoven's window was constantly open. He awaited her reply, but knew one to be impossible until Saturday. In the meantime, he tried to busy himself composing, and soon found himself sketching a piano piece inspired by Maxe's ten year old curiosity and laughter. Heaven's whitest rose, the melodies she opened! Ludwig van Beethoven was to have a daughter! On Saturday morning, there was a knock at the door. At first Beethoven did not hear it, and so the knock was repeated, growing deafeningly loud. Not Goethe again, surely! Yet more tales of famous men met that day, deliberations deliberated upon with Ambassadors, all mixed up within a cocktail of artistic theories, opinions and observations. Beethoven decided not to be in. The door knocked again, this time more softly, but with a frantic, urgent rhythm. Beethoven could hear it perfectly! And he could hear a child's voice too. He opened the door. It was Antonie. She stood there, tears streaming down her face, her hair in tatters as she anxiously and repeatedly ran her hands through its ragged curls, which framed her countenance with a look of the hunted and pursued. Her eyes were consumed by the blackest flames of Hell. "What's the matter?" said Beethoven. "Everything" said Antonie. "I'm sorry". She held out her hand. In it, was Beethoven's letter. He took it. "I can't. I just can't" she cried. Maxe looked up at Antonie bewildered. "Mummy, what is it?" Beethoven didn't need to ask. He patted Maxe on the head, and went to kiss Antonie on the cheek. She did not respond. "Do not conceal yourself from me" he said. "It's no use. I have no choice" she wept, through tears of utter confusion and torn obligations. "I am going back to Frankfurt." Beethoven could not hear her. His ears rang with confusion's rancour. "What?"

I don't like this story. I don't like it because it doesn't have a happy ending. In fact, it doesn't really have an ending at all. It just stops, unresolved. But whether you like it or not, this story could well be true. For in November 1812, Antonie Brentano left Vienna for good, and in the remaining 57 years of her long life, there's no evidence she ever returned. Neither did Beethoven ever travel to north Germany to revisit his Bonn birthplace on the Rhine, which would have given him an easy opportunity to call in on Antonie in Frankfurt on the way.

In essence, sad conclusion *et al*, the above is the story advanced by the modern Beethoven scholar Maynard Solomon. I think Solomon's story is plausible, but then Solomon is always less convincing than his surface appearance, since like many of the fusty scholars in this field, much of his erudition is really point scoring by omission. For example, Solomon implies that the finality of Beethoven and Antonie's parting in 1812 is proof the pain of reunion would have been too great. He doesn't mention that you can at least as plausibly argue that their failure to meet after 1812 simply demonstrates they didn't give a damn about each other and never had. And on top of that, Solomon's under the self-created pressure most Beethoven scholars succumb to, namely that a new book on Ludwig sells on a new candidate for the Immortal Beloved.

Well, I'm obviously no scholar because I've got no new candidates. For the record however, the major scholars fall out as follows:

SCHOLAR
IMMORTAL BELOVED

First biographer
L. Nohl
Giulietta Guicciardi
Alfred Kalischer

A.W. Thayer
M.L. La Mara
W.A.. Thomas-San Galli
Therese von Brunsvik
Romain Rolland
K. Smolle

W.A Thomas-San Galli
Amalie Sebald
(change of mind!)

Theodor von Frimmel
Magdalena Willmann

Hugo Riemann
(with reservations)

Bettina Brentano

S. Kaznelson
H. Goldschmidt
Josephine von Brunsvik

Dana Steichen
Marie Erdödy

Max Unger
Undecided (but convinced 1812)

George R. Marek
(hedging his bets)
Dorothea von Ertmann

Maynard Solomon
Antonie Brentano
(case solved!?)

In other words, experts, as ever, disagree. *Odi profanum vulgus et arceo.*

Three final reflections I make for myself. Firstly, Beethoven's punctuation is dreadful, and who ever taught him at primary school should be ashamed of themselves. Secondly, if the date of Beethoven's letter can only be right if it was written in 1795, 1801, 1807 or 1812, then I don't see why it couldn't also have been written in either 1818 or 1829, both dates when the 6th July also fell on a Monday. In both these later cases, there is *no evidence whatsoever* that Beethoven had any romantic dealings with anyone, not least because he died in 1827, but this doesn't wholly invalidate my case. It simply means that in 1818, Beethoven, a very lonely bachelor, was making the whole thing up as he went along to pass the time. Thirdly, two entire chapters of this novel would be unnecessary if Beethoven had done one of two things. He could have written the full name of his Immortal Beloved, thereby saving me and an awful lot of other people an awful lot of work (the next time you write a love letter, remember this. You never know how important it might turn out to be.) Or, if Beethoven didn't want to write her full name down (a formal practice lovers normally dispense with after all) he could at least have included the year along with the date. But then, any man who got his age wrong could easily have got the year wrong too, which would doubtless have caused just as many problems as it solved.

We end where we started. Intrigued, but not knowing, the riddle still unsolved. We know only the sentiments of the man who said this: "Unfortunately I have no wife. I found *only one*, whom no doubt I shall *never possess.*" WHO WAS SHE??!!

Michael Black

CROSSING OUT THE EMPEROR

So, he is no more than a common mortal! Now too will he tread on the rights of man, and indulge only his own ambition; now he will think himself superior to all men, and become a tyrant!, *Ludwig van Beethoven, on hearing Napoleon Bonaparte had declared himself to be the Emperor, 1804.*

Napoleon and Beethoven. Each one a name that towers in the firmament, and yet each one a prisoner, Napoleon ultimately the prisoner of St. Helena, Beethoven ultimately the prisoner of deafness. Just think, if Napoleon had stood on the exiled shores of his lonely island and screamed a scream the whole world could hear, Beethoven would still have been none the wiser. *Napoleon and Beethoven.* The two men never met, but it's as if they should have done, each one so overwhelmingly defining their own era in their chosen fields. *Napoleon and Beethoven.* The two men were the same age to within a year and both in their different ways children of the French Revolution, the former owing his career to the revolution, the latter owing to it much of his egalitarian philosophy. Napoleon Bonaparte, the ultimate riser through the ranks, and Ludwig van Beethoven, the composer as romantic genius.

Did Napoleon know that Beethoven's 3rd *Eroica* Symphony was originally dedicated to him? It is said it was the emissary of the revolutionary French Directoire, General Bernadotte, who first suggested to Beethoven the idea of a 'heroic' symphony on the subject of General Bonaparte whilst visiting Vienna in 1798. And it's an idea Beethoven obviously took to his heart.

But what we don't know is whether the Emperor Napoleon cared less when he was crossed off the dedication. And more, Beethoven was so furious upon hearing that Napoleon had crowned himself Emperor that he didn't only cross Napoleon's name out on the title page, he scratched through the paper to try and expunge any remnant of the man Beethoven considered to have betrayed the French Revolution. *The revolution was about getting rid of Emperors, not about creating new ones!* Did Napoleon even know it had happened? And if so, was he bothered? Frankly, did the Corsican Brigade General, the victor of Toulon, the victor of Montenotte, Dega, Millesima and Arcolle, the Commander-in-Chief of the campaign in Egypt, the victor of Marengo and Austerlitz, the First Consul, the Life Consul, the indomitably resolute first man of Europe..., let's face it, did the **EMPEROR***!!!* give a damn what an increasingly hard of hearing, idealistic Germanic composer thought of him? When a Viennese violinist complained the cadenza of the Violin Concerto was too difficult, Beethoven replied "what care I for the limits of your damn'd fiddling?" And so maybe Napoleon thought to himself "what care I for the dedication of your damn'd symphony?" Why should the Emperor have given a damn?

Why? Because Napoleon and Beethoven have a lot in common. And Johann Wolfgang von Goethe met both of them, so he should know. "[Beethoven's] talent amazed me" he said, adding with the fake wisdom of the self-seeking that "unfortunately he is an utterly untamed personality, who is not altogether wrong in holding the world detestable but surely does not make it any the more enjoyable either for himself or for others by his attitude." Goethe obviously didn't think Beethoven was the kind of man you took to see an Emperor, which is probably why he didn't. Goethe was very good at meeting all the right people. He was even involved in government. Perhaps governing people is what Goethe and Napoleon talked about.

Well, governing people, and Goethe's *The Sorrows of Young Werther* apparently, which the Emperor had read, and doubtless thought he could have done much better if he'd set his mind to it. The Emperor was *that kind of a guy*. If you worked for Napoleon, the one thing you never said, and I mean never ever never said, was "that is not possible." For Napoleon, the words simply didn't exist, or rather belonged "only in the dictionary of fools." Goethe said meeting him was like meeting a grand prosecutor relentlessly pursuing the defendant to the end. *Just why does young Werther commit suicide, Herr Goethe? Just what kind of a hero is that? Not much use to the Grand Armée!* Goethe also said "He was somebody and one could see that he was somebody" but I don't think that's quite right. Napoleon was somebody and he *knew he was somebody*, that's the point. And so did Beethoven. *What care I for the limits of your damn'd fiddling?* It's not my music that's the problem, it's you...

There's an attitude there, one that Napoleon would have approved of. "He was one of the most creative people ever to have lived... what matters is whether the idea, the discovery, or the deed are alive, and whether they are able to live on..." Did Goethe say that about Napoleon or about Beethoven? About Napoleon actually, but he could have said it about Beethoven. Deaf or not, Beethoven could have gone places with the Grand Armée. *If you can't do something, then get better!* If you don't know how to do something, then learn! *Nothing is impossible, and ignorance is always, always defeatable.* Who d'you think you are? *The bloody Emperor?!* And there's the rub. That's what Beethoven couldn't stand. Napoleon Bonaparte, son of a minor Corsican tax assessor, Napoleon Bonaparte, revolutionary, had declared *himself* to be the Emperor.

"Goethe delights far too much in the court atmosphere, far more than is becoming in a poet." So wrote Beethoven after meeting Goethe at Teplitz in 1812. And quite right too. You see, as far as Beethoven was concerned, you didn't acquire status, you were born with it. "Prince!" he wrote to Lichnowsky, "What you are, you are by circumstance and by birth. What I am, I am through myself. Of princes there have been and will be many thousands. Of Beethoven's there is only one." Try changing the names, and imagine saying that to your boss, or to which ever powerful person you feel like saying it to. *Say it and mean it.* Because as far as Beethoven was concerned, it represented the entire point. As far as Beethoven was concerned, we were all emperors and empresses, counts and countesses. Within each and every one of us was to be found the whole potentiality of humankind. As far as Beethoven is concerned, we are all capable of being heroes and heroines! He had to believe this to make his own life work. *He had to believe in the possibility of the deaf composer.* Beethoven spent his lifetime believing in the impossible and proving himself right. He wasn't invincible, but he knew his limitations could be overcome. Napoleon on the other hand knew of no limitations and completely failed to understand that no one is invincible. The human capacity to love and create is infinite, but so is the human capacity to self-destruct, and perhaps amongst this novel's various stories of love and war that is the most salient lesson.

Napoleon first suffered from stomach cramps in 1802. They would come on a few hours after eating, and were usually accompanied by violent physical sickness. At Austerlitz and at Wagram, at Marengo and Friedland and at Jena, at international conferences and when at home in the Elysée, the Emperor was secretly writhing in pain. He learnt to deal with it, finding light snacks of chocolate and ice cream brought much relief, and he came to carry in the inner pockets of his favourite dark-green uniform little packets of aniseed which he swallowed every time his stomach threatened further eruption. From time to time he would also faint, probably from the result of a blood sugar deficiency known as hypoglycaemia. *Some Emperor!*

And it gets worse. From 1810 onwards, the Emperor had been gradually getting fatter and fatter, to the point of downright obesity in his final years of exile. His dark-green uniform of a Colonel in the Chasseurs being now too tight, too old and too shabby, Napoleon insisted on a new one, but no suitable cloth could be found. Eventually, Hudson Lowe, the British Governor of St. Helena, ordered the old uniform be unpicked at the seams, underlaid, turned inside out and thus transformed. And transformed Napoleon certainly was. His doctor described his "beautiful hands [and] rounded breasts... Any beautiful lady might have been proud of that chest." The Emperor was turning into a woman! One recent pathologist has linked most of the above symptoms and maladies together under the Zollinger-Ellison syndromes, sufferers of which have multiple small tumours of the pancreas and over-secrete the hormone gastrin, which causes repeated ulcers to both the stomach and the duodenum. In one quarter of all patients, the gastrinoma is only one part of the disease, the other being *multiple endocrinological adenomatosis* (MEA1), a sex-linked disease resulting in tumours, often malignant, affecting the parathyroid glands as well as the pancreatic and the pituitary glands. Sufferers of MEA1 develop secondary liver and kidney disorders, as well as over producing insulin with a resultant loss in the blood sugar level. Reduced thyroid activity tends to result in obesity, fatigue, drowsiness, whiteness of skin, loss of skin hair, atrophy of the genitals and adrenal insufficiency at times of stress. In short, MEA1 has a chronic effect on both the body and the brain.

The Emperor Napoleon died a mess. And he was a mess long before his afflictions caught up with him. He was a mess because he could only ever conceive of life as one long literal battle, and inflicted his battles on everyone else. And just how many more Borodinos and Moscows do we need? How many more Sommes and Stalingrads, how many more Hiroshimas and Cambodias and Baghdads and Bazras and Vukovars and Sarajevos and Rwandas and Kosovos do we really have to impotently witness before finally on one bright and shining new day there exist enough people in one place at one time simply and strongly to say "STOP IT!" How long will it be before enough of the innocents are heard? How many more power mad Emperors will order the crossing of the Beresina whatever the cost? How many more battles will there be until then? We've all got the choice to emulate the Napoleon's of this world, or to listen to Beethoven's alternative invention of a new heroic personality that doesn't use its power and authority to dominate and kill. In Beethoven's invention of the new heroic personality of the 3rd Symphony to the triumphant exaltation of the *Ode to Joy* in the 9th is a new story of charisma, power and knowledge that understands its job is to exalt humanity, not to ride roughshod over it or dominate it. A new child is being born every day, and through that new child a new adult, and if you listen well enough to Beethoven, perhaps that new adult could still be you. In the soul of every one of us dwell the dreams of inexhaustible promise. *We are all emperors and empresses.*

Beethoven replaced his 3rd Symphony dedication to Napoleon to one which read "to the memory of a great man" emphasising the promise not the actuality of what Napoleon became. Think of Stalin. Think of Hitler or Mao. It is normally tyrants that cross out artists and many thousands and millions of others as well. Beethoven could see what was coming and got in there first. He crossed out the Emperor before the Emperor crossed him out. And the rest of us.

Crossing Out The Emperor

CAPTIVITY

After final defeat at Waterloo and in transit to exile on St. Helena:

I hereby solemnly protest, in the face of Heaven and of men, against the violence done me, and against the violation of my most sacred rights, in forcibly disposing of my person and my liberty.

I came voluntarily on board the *Bellerophon*; I am not a prisoner - I am the guest of England. I came on board at the instigation of the captain, who told me he had orders from the government to receive me and my suite, and conduct me to England, if agreeable to me. I presented myself with good faith, to put myself under the protection of the English laws. As soon as I was on board the *Bellerophon*, I was under the shelter of the British people. If the government, in giving orders to the captain of the *Bellerophon* to receive me as well as my suite, only intended to lay a snare for me, it has forfeited its honour, and disgraced its flag. If this act be consummated, the English will in vain boast to Europe of their integrity, their laws and their liberty. British good faith will be lost in the hospitality of the *Bellerophon*. I appeal to history; it will say that an enemy, who for twenty years waged war against the English people, came voluntarily, in his misfortunes, to seek asylum under their laws. What more brilliant proof could he give of his esteem and his confidence? But what return did England make for so much magnanimity? - They feigned to stretch forth a friendly hand to that enemy; and when he delivered himself up in good faith, they sacrificed him.

(Signed)   NAPOLEON
"On board *H.M.S. Bellerophon*,
4th August, 1815."

Crossing Out The Emperor

IMMORTAL BELOVED

I spent my life with my heart broken in two. I could never talk to women, or not to the women I met professionally through teaching, composing or performing, the aristocrats and acquisitive burghers of Vienna. I never found true love, but I glimpsed it. Briefly, it was like having perfect pitch.

I regret I never sent the letter. I've regretted it many times. *But I could never decide who I wanted to send it to.*

Giulietta
Therese
Josephine
Therese
Dorothea
Magdalena
Amalie
Marie
Marie
Rahel
Elise
Marie
Marie
Antonie
Bettina
Antonie

I LOVED THEM ALL

www.ingramcontent.com/pod-product-compliance
Lightning Source LLC
Chambersburg PA
CBHW020658220526
45464CB00001B/495